THE
GENESIS
DIET

THE BIBLICAL FOUNDATION
FOR OPTIMUM NUTRITION

Gordon S. Tessler, Ph. D.

DEDICATION

To my God and Father who has given me everything that pertains to life. To my Lord and Savior, Yeshua, who was and is and is to come. To my dear wife Laura, whose prayers, love, and encouragement are a constant inspiration. To all my brothers and sisters in Messiah who love the Word of God.

"Beloved I pray that you may prosper in all things and be in health, just as your soul prospers."
(3 John 2)

Table of Contents

INTRODUCTION

"Or do you not know that your body is the temple of the Holy Spirit who is in you, whom you have from God, and you are not your own? For you were bought at a price; therefore glorify God in your body."
(I Corinthians 6:19-20)

When we believe in the God of Abraham, Isaac, and Jacob and receive by faith the salvation offered at the cross of Calvary, we become a new creation (II Corinthians 5:17). As a part of this new life in Messiah, an important change takes place. Our body becomes "**the temple of the Holy Spirit.**"

So, why don't we take better care of our bodies? The answer lies in what we consider valuable. We would not dream of pouring a can of soft drink or a cup of grease on the altar at church, yet we drink cokes and eat hamburgers and fries like they are going out of style! We are so careful not to harm the church building, but we pollute the **"temple of the living God"**, our own body, as though there was no tomorrow! (II Corinthians 6: 16) We even take better care of our cars and other material possessions than we do our bodies. Material possessions have a certain value attached to them, but **our body is priceless!** God paid a great price for us, the blood of the His only Son; therefore, we need to value and take care of what God values. Learning to follow the Lord's instructions about the care of our temple is the purpose of **The Genesis Diet.**

7

LACK OF KNOWLEDGE

One of the primary reasons for the epidemic levels of heart disease, strokes, cancer, arthritis, diabetes, and obesity in America today is poor nutrition. For the average American, everything that is edible is food but to God, only those things which He calls "food" are edible. The poisoned, processed, and devitalized foods that make up the Standard American Diet (S.A.D.) are destroying the next generation as well as the present one. No wonder that the number one prayer in most congregations today is for healing - healing for ourselves, our family members, and our friends. In the history of the church, there have never been more healing ministries, books and tapes about healing, or opportunities for elders to pray for the sick than now, yet the body of Messiah continues to be afflicted with every known illness and disease. Why? We lack the knowledge of God's word on the subject of Biblical nutrition and how to implement, or sow, these principles into our lives in order to reap the health our Creator intended for us. The Bible says in Hosea:

"My people are destroyed for lack of knowledge.
......you have forgotten the law (the instructions)*
of your God,"
(Hosea 4: 6)

The God of the universe **is** interested in what His creatures eat and He has specific nutritional principles for the care of our temple because He wants us to live a long, healthy life.

GOD ESTABLISHES PRINCIPLES

God has set in motion certain physical principles (laws or rules). The law of gravity is one example of God's natural or physical principles. You can't see gravity or touch it, yet if you jump off the Empire State Building you come face to face with the tragic cost of breaking such a law. Whether you "believe" in gravity or deny its existence, God's physical principle of gravity still influences your life. Similarly, the nutritional principles found in the Scriptures influence your health whether you believe in them or not. Violators of these nutritional principles most of the time will pay a terrible price in pain, suffering, and premature death. Present day cultures in other parts of the world who have knowingly or unknowingly eaten in accordance with Biblical nutritional principles experience little or no degenerative disease even in today's poisoned environment. Individuals in these extraordinarily healthy cultures live full, energetic lives well into their 80's, 90's, and even beyond 100 years of age demonstrating that God's health principles work!

THE ULTIMATE NUTRITIONIST

God created and designed us; therefore, only He knows our complete chemical make-up down to the minutest atom and what we must eat to be healthy. David said of the Lord:

"Your hands have made me and fashioned me;"

(Psalm 119: 73)

Nutrition books with their various and contradictory man-made philosophies of eating create a spirit of confusion in the minds of many. Man's philosophies change but God's word does not change (Malachi 3: 6). We must return to the Bible, the revealed word of God, to restore the health and vitality our Creator intended for us to have.

The Bible instructs us how to live in this life and how to prepare for eternity.

B-stands for **Basic**
I-stands for **Instructions**
B-stands for **Before**
L-stands for **Leaving**
E-stands for **Earth**

The most complete, most nutritious diet for man can be found in the Bible. From Genesis to Revelation God gives His people nutritional instructions. For instance, shortly after the Israelites were delivered out of Egypt by the hand of Almighty God, He made fundamental changes in their diet. Our Lord is well aware that nutrition plays an important part in the physical, mental, emotional, and spiritual well being of man. **Following God's instructions on nutrition are not a requirement for entering heaven but they are necessary for our physical welfare while we live on earth.**

WATCH OVER OUR FLESH

Many believers feel that paying too much attention to the needs of the body is caring more for the flesh rather than the spirit. Yet, the Bible clearly teaches that we are triune beings - **spirit, soul, and body** (I Thessalonians 5: 23). To God, **the body is a temple** (I Corinthians 6: 19) and **the body is holy** (I Corinthians 3:17). In Romans 12: 1 the apostle Paul urges us to **"present your bodies a living and holy sacrifice, acceptable to God, which is your spiritual service of worship."** Therefore, the motivation for eating healthy is to glorify God in our body (I Corinthians 6:20) rather than to gratify our flesh. Our carnal nature or flesh leads us away from God's foods and tempts us to indulge in unhealthy foods. Even Jesus encourages us to watch over our flesh.

"Watch and pray, lest you enter into temptation.
The spirit is willing, but the flesh is weak."
(Matthew 26: 41)

When we feed our bodies according to God's prescribed foods, it is an act of obedience to the Spirit, rather than the desires of the flesh, and it brings Him glory. By obeying His commandments we demonstrate our love for God. The Lord commanded us to be well and He gave us a statute of health to follow.

STATUTE OF HEALTH

To walk in divine health is a **blessing** and to suffer with sickness is a **curse.** Throughout the Bible, sickness and disease is always a curse and health is always a blessing. In fact, health is not only a blessing in the Bible, health is a statute. A statute is a law and it is a promise.

After the Lord parted the Red Sea for the children of Israel and they walked through on dry ground, He led them into the wilderness. After three days in the wilderness, they found no water, except the bitter waters of Marah. The Lord showed Moses a tree which he threw into the waters and the waters became sweet. After this great miracle, the Lord makes health a law:

"There He made a statute and a law for them. And there He tested them, and said, 'If you diligently heed the voice of the Lord your God and do what is right in His sight, give ear to His commandments and keep all His statutes, I will put none of the

11

diseases on you which I have brought on the Egyptians. For I am the Lord who heals you.' "

(Exodus 15: 25-26)

Many of us only quote the last sentence of this verse, "For I am the Lord who heals you", without realizing that **this promise from God is conditional**. The four conditions that God lists are summed up in the phrase, **"do what is right in His sight"**. If we do, we are promised healing and not only healing, but more importantly, God will not put or permit disease to come upon us! **God's concern extends beyond the healing of disease to the prevention of disease!** Supernatural intervention by God to heal us of sickness or disease is wonderful, but that is not God's best. Walking in divine health, free of sickness and disease is His best for us! This profound truth is available to every believer, but because we have not been taught this divine truth, many are looking for healing from the Lord rather than health.

God often repeats Himself, especially when He wants to get an important truth across. The promise of divine health is repeated again in Exodus 23:25:

"So you shall serve the Lord your God, and He will bless your bread and water. And I will take sickness away from the midst of you."

(Exodus 23: 25)

The Lord promises that if we serve Him, He will bless our food and bless us with divine health. The Lord says that in the mouth of two or three witnesses every word is established (II Corinthians 13:1) and thus we find God repeating His promise of divine health a third time:

"And the Lord will take away from you every sickness, and will afflict you with none of the terrible diseases of Egypt which you have known, but will lay them on all those who hate you."

(Deuteronomy 7: 15)

And finally, we have the true and faithful witness, Jesus, who not only took upon Himself our sins, but also our sicknesses. Jesus, by His atonement on the cross, bore our sins and sicknesses; therefore, we do not have to bear them. **We can walk in divine health.**

"...And He cast out the spirits with a word, and healed all who were sick, that it might be fulfilled which was spoken by Isaiah the prophet, saying, 'He Himself took our infirmities and bore our sicknesses.' "

(Matthew 8: 16-17)

The Lord made divine health a statute and confirmed it at the cross. He commands us to be well! Whoever would ask for the blessing of divine health must do those things which are right in the sight of God and not those which are right in his own sight (Judges 21:25). Unfortunately, Adam and Eve chose to do what was right in their own sight, forgetting the commandment of God.

THE FIRST SIN

God gave the first man and woman many wonderful and delicious foods which He set apart or sanctified for them to enjoy and commanded them to eat only those foods. A commandment which they broke. **The first sin committed by man was not murder or adultery or stealing; it was eating something they were told not to eat!** And man has been eating things he shouldn't eat ever since. This present age is witnessing the dulling of man's senses to distinctions between right and wrong - good and evil. But we possess the power to choose to follow God and receive the blessing of divine health.

"I set before you life and death, blessing and cursing; therefore choose life, that both you and your descendants may live;"
(Deuteronomy 30: 19)

The Genesis Diet will teach you what God, our Creator, has to say about nutrition. His principles for optimum nutrition are as valuable today as they were thousands of years ago! After all, who knows better what we must eat to be healthy than He who created us! And as we walk in His precepts for optimum health, we are freed from sickness and disease that plagues mankind.

"And I walk at liberty (in a wide place), For I seek your precepts."
(Psalm 119: 45)

*The Hebrew word **Torah** was translated into the Greek word **nomos** meaning **law.** However, the Hebrew word **Torah** does not mean **law** but means **" the teaching"** or **"the instruction"** of God. The word **(instructions)** was added to Hosea 4:6 by the author to emphasize the point that we are perishing because we do not know the instructions or the teachings of God regarding Biblical nutrition.

CHAPTER ONE

DECEPTIVE FOODS

"When you sit down to eat with a ruler, consider carefully what is before you; and put a knife to your throat if you are a man given to appetite. Do not desire his delicacies, for they are deceptive foods".
(Proverbs 23: 1-3)

Many times appetite rather than hunger causes us to desire and eat foods that are not good for us. There is a tremendous difference between true hunger and appetite. Hunger is a necessary urge that forces us to eat in order to live. Hunger is a God-given desire for man's physical survival and we should direct our hunger toward the foods God prescribed for us to eat. Only the foods our Creator directed for us to eat will satisfy the biological urge to replenish the body's nutritional needs. Hunger may be satisfied while appetite persists. Appetite causes us to overindulge (gluttony) in food and to desire foods that God has not recommended. Hunger is triggered by the biological need for food while appetite is a craving triggered by the sight, taste, smell, or even thought of food. After a meal, no man is hungry when he reaches for dessert!

The Bible warns us that our appetite will cause us to crave a ruler's delicacies and that these delicacies are "deceptive foods". Rulers and kings ate the richest, most fattening foods that money could buy. These foods looked good and tasted good, but they were full of animal fat and sugar that led to a long list of what was referred to as the "king's diseases" - heart disease, cancer, strokes, diabetes, arthritis, and obesity. Only the rich could afford to eat much meat or buy refined sugar. It was a luxury to use land to graze a few cattle to feed a few people while the same land could grow grains, beans, fruits, and vegetables to feed many people. The peasants ate beans while the rich ate meat. Today, the diet of our entire culture is based upon a ruler's delicacies. Since the Standard American Diet (S.A.D.) consists mostly of these "deceptive foods", America leads all other nations in the development of degenerative diseases. The idea that a food could look good and taste good, yet be destructive did not begin in America or kings' palaces.

APPETITE OF ADAM AND EVE

The first deceptive food was eaten back in the garden of Eden. God set apart or sanctified many wonderful and delicious foods for Adam and Eve to enjoy and satisfy their biological hunger, but He also commanded them to stay away from a certain tree.

"but of the tree of the knowledge of good and evil you shall not eat, for in the day that you eat of it you shall surely die."

(Genesis 2 : 17)

Two statements can be made about God's heart towards man:

1. God wanted man to know only good and not evil. Up until the time that Adam and Eve sinned, man only knew God and God is "good". God's heart was to protect man so that he would only know Him and be spared the pain of knowing evil. God knew that knowing evil meant coming to know the author of evil, the devil himself.

2. God wanted man to live and not die. God is the Creator of all living things and He brings life abundantly! Satan is a murderer who comes to steal, and to kill, and to destroy.

Adam and Eve heard God's instructions about what to eat and not to eat but they were tempted by evil and enticed by their own desire or appetite for that which was **not good** for them. After giving in to temptation, Eve admits to God, "The serpent **deceived** me, and I ate."(Genesis 3:13) The words **deception, deceive, and deceit** all have the same meaning - **making a person believe as true something that is false.** The serpent convinced Eve that the food from the tree of the knowledge of good and evil would not harm her. Eve, like so many after her, didn't realize how dangerous it can be to eat something that God commands not to eat. The deception that took place in the garden concerning forbidden foods is still with us today. Our natural hunger for food is being exploited by a deceptive spirit that tempts us away from God's wholesome and necessary foods.

DECEPTIVE ADVERTISING

The first deceptive advertising about food was done by satan in the garden of Eden, a beautiful, natural setting, as Eve looked at this cocky serpent giving her the false impression that this forbidden fruit would not harm her. Imagine this picture: The serpent standing near or even sitting in the forbidden tree, perhaps holding a piece of the forbidden fruit, and Eve, seeing this, says to herself, "the serpent hasn't been hurt by touching this so-called dangerous food and I won't be either!"

So many television commercials are full of the same deception that Eve experienced at the hand of the serpent. The advertisers appeal to our senses and our emotions - it tastes good, it looks good, and it won't harm you! These commercials depict healthy young people having a "great time" in a "natural setting" while they are drinking beer, smoking cigarettes, eating junk food, or sipping their favorite can of soft drink. The association the advertisers want us to make is that these attractive, healthy young people are not harmed by these products. The television viewer thinks, "See how healthy and happy they are! These products won't harm me because they haven't harmed them!" Wrong! The advertisers neglect to mention how many deaths are caused by drinking and driving or how many heart attacks and other degenerative diseases are caused by high fat, high sugar junk foods. Most of the "beautiful young people" in these commercials are actors and models that starve themselves to "look good". They work out for hours each day in a gym and probably don't use the products they promote. Have you noticed that God's wholesome foods are rarely advertised? **If you never eat or drink anything advertised on television you will probably be very healthy!**

DECEPTIVE WORDS

Besides the deceptive picture Eve was seeing, the serpent's deceptive words tempted her to disobey God's command. The serpent said three things to Eve about the

Word of God that are still being said by many today:

    1. **Doubt the Word of God** - "Has God indeed said, 'you shall not eat of every tree of the garden'?" (Genesis 3:1) Satan, the author of confusion, caused Eve to question God's commandment.

    2. **Deny the Word of God** - "You will not surely die." (Genesis 3:4) With this statement, satan, the father of lies, replaces the truth of God's word with a lie.

    3. **Defy the Word of God** - "For God knows that in the day you eat of it your eyes will be opened, and you will be like God, knowing good and evil." (Genesis 3:5) Satan, destroyed God's authority in Eve's eyes and tempted her to think that she could be as wise as God.

THREE DEADLY DESIRES

    Satan encouraged Eve to focus on her own needs and desires rather than the commandment and provision of God. She became self-centered not God-centered. After seeing and hearing the serpent, Eve made three justifications for eating the forbidden fruit.

"So the woman saw that the tree was good for food, that it was pleasant to the eyes, and a tree desirable to make one wise, she took of its fruit and ate. She also gave to her husband with her, and he ate."

(Genesis 3:6)

Eve saw that the tree was:

    1. **"good for food"**-The appeal was to her **appetite** and she was drawn away from the

commandment of God by her own desire to taste the fruit. Appetite not controlled by the Word of God gives way to the lust of the flesh.

2. **"pleasant to the eyes"**-She saw something **attractive** and that attraction, caused her to say in her heart "I want that". Unrestrained by the Word of God, she yielded to the lust of the eyes, which is also known as coveting.

3. **"desirable to make one wise"**- She placed her desire for wisdom above the wisdom of God not realizing that the beginning of wisdom is the fear or reverence of the Lord. By taking her eyes off God and focusing on her own desire for wisdom, Eve yielded to the pride of life. And God opposes the proud. We can only possess God's wisdom when we obey God's word.

In **I John 2:16** the Apostle John calls these three observations made by the "First Lady" Eve, a worldly and temporary view of existence.

"For all that is in the world....the lust of the flesh, the lust of the eyes, and the pride of life....is not of the Father but is of the world. And the world is passing away, and the lust of it; but he who does the will of God abides forever."
(I John 2: 16)

LUST FOR FOOD

We don't often equate lust with food. But whether we **crave** unhealthy sex or unhealthy food, it's all carnality. Desiring or lusting after food, other than what God has given, brings destruction. Scripture tell us that the children of Israel were not satisfied with the manna, a life-sustaining grain, that God had provided for them. They complained to Moses that they were hungry for meat. Numbers 11 tells us that they **"wept in the hearing of the Lord, saying, "Who will give us meat to eat? For it was well with us in Egypt"**. Verse 4 says that the Israelites "**yielded to intense craving"** and this displeased God. The Lord provided the meat which they craved in the form of quail, but afterwards He also struck them with a great plague.

"But while the meat was still between their teeth, before it was chewed......the Lord struck the people with a very great plague......they buried the people who had yielded to craving."
(Numbers 11:34-35)

Many people in this country have an "intense craving" for the modern "flesh pots of Egypt" rather than being satisfied with the wholesome, nourishing foods which God has provided. Fast food restaurants today are not attracting millions of customers by serving whole grains and green vegetables. These modern "flesh pots" serve processed foods which are high in animal fat and low in nutritional value.

DECEPTIVE FOODS TODAY

Today the food processing industry makes billions of dollars a year trying to make foods better than the original. The spirit behind this deception is none other that satan himself. Just as Eve was deceived into believing that she could be as wise as God, man believes that he has the wisdom to improve upon the taste and appearance of the natural, wholesome foods that God created. Although processed foods may look good, taste good, and promise to "build strong bodies twelve ways", these foods are truly deceptive foods. They look like the real thing but they are not! Many of the "foods" we consume have imitation flavors and colors and the nutritional value has been removed. These deceptive foods may fool your taste buds but they do not fulfill the nutritional needs of your body. **Processed foods are just cheap imitations; full of refined sugar, greasy fat, synthetic vitamins, and air.** These lifeless, empty calorie, junk foods are the primary cause of cancer, heart disease, diabetes, arthritis, and obesity in the United States.

Modern processing began in the United States back in the 1940's. The purpose of "processing" any food was to extend its shelf life. Food processors are not concerned with **your life** but with **shelf life**. For example, by removing the bran and germ of wheat, the flour can be made into bread that will not spoil as quickly. However, in removing the bran and the germ, twenty-two vitamins and minerals are also removed! Scientific studies in the 1940's demonstrated that this processed flour was causing B-1, B-2, B-3 and iron deficiencies in the American population. The United States Congress passed **The Enrichment Act** of 1948 that forced food processors to add these four nutrients back into the flour they **"refined"**. The word "refined" means "free from impurities". God creates a whole grain called wheat containing bran, wheat germ, plus twenty-two vitamins and minerals and man calls them **"impurities"** and removes them! The labels on these "wonderful" breads reads **"ENRICHED"**! What deceptive words! What arrogance! The word "arrogance" is defined as "a disposition or character to make exorbitant claims of rank, dignity, or estimation; the pride which exalts one's own importance". This definition certainly applies to most advertising today!

DEN OF THIEVES

When Jesus entered the temple in Jerusalem and threw out the money changers He said:

"My house is a house of prayer, but you have made it a den of thieves."

(Luke 19:46, Matthew 21:13, Mark 11:17)

The temple made with hands has been replaced by the temple made by God, our body. The vast majority of the foods that Americans put in their bodies have been "processed" or maybe a better word would be **"destroyed"** by the arrogance of man who takes the foods of God and alters them to suit his tastes, whims, and greed. These processed foods are not only destroyed but can also destroy our bodies as well. There are four "white deaths", as nutritionists call them, that rob us of our life:

1. White salt

Processed table salt with added inorganic iodine is 99% sodium chloride and the average American eats 10 times the bodily requirement. **Overconsumption of salt depletes your body of potassium.** Without enough potassium, symptoms such as loss of memory, mental confusion, water retention, weight gain, and heart palpitations may be experienced. Excessive salt consumption can overwork your kidneys! There is plenty of natural sodium in God's foods without adding any; however, if you must add salt, 500 milligrams (1/4 teaspoon) of sea salt a day is the limit!

2. White sugar

Sugar cane and sugar beets are full of vitamins, minerals, fiber, and about 15% sucrose or sugar.

After these natural sugars are processed all the vitamins, minerals and fiber are gone and what's left is 95% sucrose!

White sugar robs your cells of needed oxygen. White sugar overworks your pancreas and uses up too much insulin. Overconsumption of white sugar over many years can damage the insulin mechanism and can lead to diabetes (lack of adequate insulin production). All sugars, whether natural or refined, require B-complex, calcium and magnesium to aid in their digestion. Natural sugars like grains, fruits, and vegetables contain enough of these important nutrients to assist the body in their own digestion. Refined sugar like white sugar removes these and many other precious vitamins and minerals. Your body must take B-complex from your nervous system and calcium/magnesium from your bones to digest refined sugars. Because white sugar depletes the nervous system of B-complex, nerves become "raw". One of the leading causes of osteoporosis (thinning bones) is the overuse of white sugar which forces the body to take calcium/magnesium out of the bones. **The average American eats 120 to 150 pounds of white sugar a year!**

3. White flour

Today we eat bread from which twenty-two naturally-occuring vitamins and minerals have been systematically removed and four synthetic nutrients have been added (see Enrichment Act of 1948 above). Not only are most of the body-building nutrients gone, but most of the commercial breads add white sugar, white salt, and fat!

4. White fat

Time-trend data for the United States shows that the percent of fat in the American diet increased from 32% to 43% between 1915 and 1985. On a yearly basis, this increase is equal to 24 pounds of fat per person! The reason why so many Americans are overweight is simple—they eat too much fat! Much of the fat consumed is high cholesterol, saturated fat which contributes to coronary heart disease, strokes, and cancer. Saturated fats are primarily found in animal products such as meats, dairy products, and eggs.

Americans have significantly increased their consumption of polyunsaturated vegetable oils in an effort to cut both cholesterol and saturated fat from their diets. However, the overwhelming majority of these vegetable oils are in the form of hardened vegetable fat! Hydrogenation or hardening vegetable oils allows a manufacturer to buy a cheap vegetable oil and transform it into a product that can compete with butter. Margarine, is an example of one of these man-made fats called trans-fats. These trans-fats can actually contribute to cardiovascular disease, raise cholesterol levels, and inhibit normal essential fatty acid metabolism. Americans need to reduce the amount of fat in their diet from 43% (mostly animal origin) to 15% (mostly vegetable fat without hydrogenation).

It's time we stop putting into our temples the foods that rob us of the health God wants us to have. It's time to throw the money changers out of our temple! We can choose to say "no" to the "white thieves" of sugar, salt, flour, and fat, and say "yes" to the healthy ways of the Lord.

CHOOSE HIS WAY

Our choice is between processed, man-made foods and wholesome, God-made foods. Man-made foods bring sickness and premature death while God's foods nourish and strengthen our bodies to live a long life. We can make a decision to follow God's rules concerning proper nutrition no matter what our food cravings are and by the power of the Holy Spirit, we can resist temptation. The word "genesis" means beginning and the Book of Genesis establishes God's dietary regime for man - the foods essential for optimum health. God has the answer—eat **The Genesis Diet**!

"Feed me with the food You prescribe for me;"
(Proverbs 30:8C)

CHAPTER TWO

BACK TO THE GARDEN
(GOD'S PERFECT DIET)

"And God said, 'See, I have given you every herb
that yields seed which is on the face of all the
earth, and every tree whose fruit yields seed;
to you it shall be for food.' "
Genesis 1:29

In the "Book of Beginnings", Genesis, God created man
in His own image, after His likeness, and told him what to
eat.   The Lord showed Adam and Eve the wholesome,
beautiful foods that He had created for them and said "**I
have given you**" these foods. Furthermore, He commanded the man and the woman to eat these life-sustaining foods when He said **"to you it <u>shall</u> be for food"**.
These seed-bearing plants and trees are the foundation of
God's perfect diet for man and God called them good.

"And the earth brought forth grass, the herb (plant)
that yields seed according to its kind, and the tree
that yields fruit, whose seed is in itself according to
its kind. And God saw that it was good."
(Genesis 1:12)

FREELY EAT

Many doctors, nutritionists, dieticians, and weight loss centers have taught us to "limit" our calories if we want to stay slim and healthy; but counting calories and calorie restriction is a man-made doctrine, not a commandment of God. In fact, the Lord tells us to **"freely eat"** (without limit) of the foods that He has given to us. In the second chapter of Genesis, the Lord establishes this very important principle of nutrition.

"Then the Lord commanded the man, saying, 'Of every tree of the garden you may freely eat; but of the tree of the knowledge of good and evil you shall not eat, for in the day that you eat of it you shall surely die".

(Genesis 2: 16-17)

The Lord wanted man to choose only the food which He had given and called good and forsake the food that may look good or even taste good but its end for us is death. From the beginning, we see the love of our Creator as He cared for the nutritional needs of His creation.

SEEDS: IDEAL ENERGY SOURCE

The **"seed-bearing herbs or plants"** and the **"trees whose fruit yield seed"** include any edible food in the vegetable kingdom that can reproduce itself. All life on this earth either eats the plants grown from seed or eats the animals that have eaten the plants of these powerful seeds. **That is why God, our Father, made them of prime importance for Adam and Eve.** The nutritional program that God introduced in the Garden of Eden was a high fiber, high complex carbohydrate, low protein, low fat, low sodium vegetarian diet. So God was the first to say "Eat your vegetables. They are good for you!" **These "seed-bearing plants" include the following food groups:**

> **1. Grains, beans, and legumes**
> **2. Nuts and Seeds**
> **3. Vegetables**
> **4. Fruits**
> **5. Herbs and Spices**

Seed-bearing plants and trees were designed (by you know who!) for immediate and long-term energy requirements. The starch or endosperm portion of a seed is a pure carbohydrate energy source called **glucose**. Glucose is another name for **God's natural sugar.** Glucose is the fuel needed to run every cell in our body as well as most bodily functions including the brain, nerves, and muscles.

Grains are complex carbohydrates that provide the longest-lasting form of natural sugar among the seed-bearing plants. These complex carbohydrates also contain important vitamins, minerals, fiber, phytochemicals, and chlorophyll. Human beings have lived primarily on complex carbohydrates for thousands of years. Without an abundant supply of complex carbohydrates (seed-bearing plants) in our diet, there would not be sufficient energy to live, work, or enjoy life. How magnificent and powerful is the energy packed into a plant seed! A seed contains all the genetic information to reproduce after its own kind and most seeds reproduce hundreds of seeds from a single seed!

MAKE-UP OF A KERNEL OF GRAIN
Oats, brown rice, millet, barley, buckwheat, rye, cornmeal.

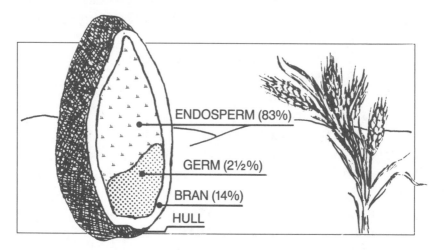

ENDOSPERM (83%)

GERM (2½%)

BRAN (14%)

HULL

TOTAL NUTRIENTS IN A KERNEL OF GRAIN

GERM	BRAN	ENDOSPERM
Thiamine (B^1) Riboflavin (B^2) Pyridoxine (B^6) Protein Pantothenic Acid (B^5) Niacin (B^3) Vitamin E	Pyridoxine (B^6) Pantothenic Acid (B^5) Riboflavin (B^2) Thiamine (B^1) Protein	Starch Traces of Vitamins & Minerals

MINERALS

Calcium	Sulphur	Barium
Iron	Iodine	Silver
Phosphorus	Fluorine	Inositol
Magnesium	Chlorine	Folic Acid
Potassium	Sodium	Choline
Manganese	Silicon	And other trace
Copper	Boron	materials

Source: Nutrition Almanac

The grains, beans, legumes, nuts, seeds, vegetables, and fruits are a treasure chest of vitality and energy, unequaled in the food kingdom. **The sparks of life and nourishment placed by our Creator in the seeds of plants are of supreme importance for man's physical life, his health, his virility, and his energy.**

POWER OF GREEN

Scientific research has "discovered" that chlorophyll, the green-colored matter in plants, has almost the exact molecular structure of hemoglobin in human blood. Chlorophyll in the plants we eat helps build healthy blood in humans by supplying the blood with oxygen, nutrients, and phytochemicals (compounds in plants that protect our body against cancer and other diseases). Green grasses and green plants are rich sources of such important nutrients as beta-carotenes, antioxidants, digestible proteins, and fiber which help to sustain and protect us from illness and disease.

Through photosynthesis, plants convert sunshine into chemical energy. Photosynthesis is the process by which plant cells make carbohydrates from carbon dioxide and water in the presence of chlorophyll and sunlight. Some scientists believe that photosynthesis is the most important chemical reaction in nature because man depends upon plants to gather the sun energy and make it available to us as food. A plant only uses about one-sixth of the sun energy it captures to sustain itself. The remaining five-sixths is stored in chemical bonds, ready for human metabolism to break it down into useful energy. **This solar energy captured and stored by plants as carbohydrates and then released by the metabolism of humans makes all the work of the body possible.**

PLANT PROTEIN

Protein consists of 22 amino acids connected in chains. The length and sequence of the amino acids distinguishes one type of protein from another type. Of the 22 amino acids, nine can not be produced within the body (essential amino acids) and therefore, must be included in your diet. Although the quantity of amino acids in plant protein is lower than animal sources, **plants are not missing any of the 22 amino acids**. The real standard of protein is the quality, not quantity of the amino acids. Quality refers to usability of the protein. **If plant and animal protein are compared in terms of quality, there is little difference between the two classes of proteins.** The **grains**, **beans, legumes, nuts, seeds, vegetables, and fruits** not only provide excellent protein but cholesterol-free fats and high fiber as well. **Isn't God a great provider!**

ESSENTIAL AMINO ACID CONTENT per 100 grams (3½ oz.)									
	in milligrams								
	TRYPTO-PHAN	THREO-NINE	ISOLEU-CINE	LEU-CINE	LYSINE	METH-IONINE	PHENY-LALANINE	VALINE	HISTI-DINE	PROTEIN GRAMS
GRAINS									
BARLEY	160	433	545	889	433	184	661	643	239	8.2
CORN (field whl)	61	398	462	1,296	288	186	454	510	206	8.9
MILLET	248	456	635	1,746	383	270	506	682	240	9.9
RICE, brown	81	294	352	646	296	135	377	524	126	7.5
RYE, whl grain	137	448	515	813	494	191	571	631	276	12.1
LEGUMES									
PINTO BEANS	213	997	1,306	1,976	1,708	232	1,270	1,395	655	22.9
LENTILS	216	896	1,316	1,760	1,528	180	1,104	1,360	548	24.7
NUTS/SEEDS									
ALMONDS	176	610	873	1,454	582	259	1,146	1,124	514	18.6
PECANS	138	389	553	773	435	153	564	525	273	9.2
SUNFLOWER	343	911	1,276	1,736	868	443	1,220	1,354	586	24.0

Source: Amino Acid Content of Foods, Home Economics Research Report #4, U.S. Department of Agriculture, 1968.

The protein content of plant foods is more than adequate to fulfill and maintain the body's requirements for protein. In Scriptural fact, the first and preferred diet for man and beast, commanded by God, was a vegetarian diet. Dairy products, fish, poultry, and red meats do not come from seed-bearing plants and are not mentioned in **Genesis 1:29.** Even though the fish were swimming in pure, clean oceans and streams and the eggs, dairy products, birds, and animals were free of antibiotics, steroids, and artificial hormones, God did not include them in His garden diet. Our Creator intended for man and beast to live in a beautiful garden and be vegetarians. Even after man was driven out of the garden, men of God continued to include in their diets the seed-bearing plants commanded in Genesis 1:29. The seed-bearing plants are God's best for man's nutritional welfare and grains are at the top of His list.

MANNA: WHAT IS IT?

The Creator of the universe could have provided any food He wanted to feed the children of Israel in the wilderness. He could have provided T-bone steaks, hamburgers and french fries, ice cream or chocolate. Instead He selected the one food which was nutritionally complete, high in fiber, and high in natural sugar:

"And the house of Israel called its name manna.

And it was like white coriander seed, and the taste

of it was like wafers made with honey."

(Exodus 16:31)

God did not give the fatted calf as food, but He gave the **life-sustaining power of seeds** as He had done in the garden diet. God gave His children a seed or grain that would provide the nourishment they would need to walk forty years in the wilderness while they lived in tents. He knew that seeds of grain would provide their

bodies balanced nutrition and give them physical strength
for the long journey. The children of Israel made por-
ridge, bread, and pastry cakes out of this seed and it
sustained the young and the old very well (Numbers 11:8).
The Israelites called God's grain, **manna**, which means in
the Hebrew language, "**what is it?**".

*"So when the children of Israel saw it, they said to
one another, "What is it?' For the did not know
what it was. And Moses said to them, "This is the
bread which the Lord has given you to eat.' "*
(Exodus 16:15)

Many people today, when presented with barley, buckwheat, lentils or millet, will make a face and say, "Eck,
what is it and what do I do with it?" Let us not be like the
stiff-necked, rebellious children of Israel who were spoiled
by the "delicacies" of decadent Egypt. May we, His children, appreciate God's seed-bearing plants which He
intended for us to eat from the very beginning.

JOSEPH STORED GRAIN

As second in command, Joseph prepared for the seven
years of famine foretold by God in Pharaohs dream (Genesis 41:29-30) by storing grain:

*"And let them gather all the food of those good
years that are coming, and store up grain under the
authority of Pharaoh,...."*
(Genesis 41:35)

Just as manna, a grain, kept the Israelites well for
forty years in the wilderness, we see that grain (the life-
sustaining power of seeds) was used again to provide for

the nutritional needs of the people during the seven years of famine.

DANIEL'S EXPERIMENT

Daniel, the great prophet who was given a prophetic vision of the end times (Daniel 9:24-27), also knew the **power of seed-bearing plants.** King Nebuchadnezzar, after taking Jerusalem, brought the brightest of Israel's young men into his palace in Babylon. Daniel was one of these gifted young men. They were taught the language and the literature of the Chaldeans and given the best food available in Babylon — directly from king Nebuchadnezzer's table. But Daniel understood the importance of eating God's foods rather than the deceptive foods of a ruler:

"But Daniel purposed in his heart that he would not defile himself with the portion of the king's delicacies, nor with the wine which he drank; therefore he requested of the chief of the eunuches that he might not defile himself."

(Daniel 1:8)

Daniel had come into favor with the chief of the eunuchs, but the chief was afraid to let Daniel eat anything besides what the king had recommended:

"I fear my lord the king, who has appointed your food and drink. For why should he see your faces looking worse than the young men who are your

age? Then you would endanger
my head before the king."
(Daniel 110)

The chief of the eunuchs believed, as so many do today, that anyone who eats just grains, vegetables, and fruits will endanger their health and could not possibly be as healthy as some who eat meat (the food of kings!). But Daniel knew the truth about seed-bearing plants and designed one of the first nutritional experiments ever done:

"Please test your servants for ten days, and let
them give us vegetables and water to drink. Then
let our countenances be examined before you, and
the countenances of the young men who eat the
portion of the king's delicacies; and as you see fit,
so deal with your servants."
(Daniel 1:12-13)

So a test was designed by the prophet Daniel to see which diet was better: a vegetable diet or a meat diet. The results were so dramatic, **as they will be with you,** that permanent changes were instituted:

"And at the end of ten days their countenance
appeared better and fatter in flesh than all the
young men who ate the portion of the king's delica-
cies. Thus the steward took away their portion of
the delicacies and the wine that they were to drink,

and gave them vegetables."

(Daniel 1:15-16)

EZEKIEL'S BREAD

The great prophet Ezekiel knew the importance of eating sufficient quantities of grains, vegetables, seeds, nuts, and fruit for optimum health. Ezekiel was told by God to exclusively eat grains for 390 days:

"Also take for yourself wheat, barley, beans, lentils, millet, and spelt; put them into one vessel, and make bread of them for yourself. During the number of days that you lie on your side, three hundred and ninety days, you shall eat it."

(Ezekiel 4:9)

Do you think the Lord would have told the great prophet Ezekiel to eat only plant foods if it would have been unhealthy for him to do so?

JACOB'S GRAIN STEW

Esau, the brother of Jacob, sold his birthright to his brother for a serving of homebaked bread and a delicious bowl of lentil stew!

"And Jacob gave Esau bread and stew of lentils; then he ate and drank, arose, and went his way. Thus Esau despised his birthright."

(Genesis 25:34)

At least Esau had a taste for healthy seed-bearing plants. Today, many people sell their precious gift of health for a hamburger and fries!

THE LORD'S HOLY DAYS

God's Holy Feast Days in Leviticus 23 are based on the harvesting of grains. Passover and Unleaven Bread revolve around eating unleavened bread for seven days. The Feast of Firstfruits celebrates the barley harvest which the priest waves before the Lord. The Feast of Pentecost celebrates the spring wheat harvest and the priest waves two loaves of leavened wheat bread before the Lord. The Feast of Tabernacle is a celebration of the ingathering of the fall harvest of wheat and other produce from the field.

GRAIN OFFERING

The Lord made provision for the Tabernacle and later, the Temple in Jerusalem, for the priests and the people to give a grain offering to Him. A grain offering could be of fine flour mixed with olive oil or unleavened cakes mixed with oil. But regardless of the type of grain offering:

"It is a most holy offering of the offerings to the Lord made with fire."

(Leviticus 2: 3)

The grain offering was considered "most holy" to God. The greatest grain offering of all, Yeshua, referred to Himself as "the Bread of Life" (John 6:48) and also as a "grain of wheat" (John 12:24). Jesus also performed great miracles with the five barley loaves (Matthew 14:17, Luke 9:13, John 6:90).

SHEDDING OF BLOOD

After banishment from the garden, the ancestors of Adam and Eve continued to be vegetarians until the time of the flood. However, the killing of animals for use as sacrifices started after Adam and Eve disobeyed God's command not to eat of the tree of the knowledge of good and evil. Adam and Eve's sin caused God himself to shed the first blood of an innocent animal for sin and gave the animal skins to them:

"Also for Adam and his wife the Lord God made tunics of skin, and clothed them."

(Genesis 3:21)

And from the time that Adam and Eve sinned, the worshippers of God sacrificed clean animals to acknowledge their sins before Him (Genesis 4:4, 8:20). The blood of an animal was required when man sinned against God until the final and complete sacrifice was made by Jesus on the cross of Calvary.

THE GARDEN DIET:
FOUNDATION FOR OPTIMUM HEALTH

The garden of Eden had varieties of seed-bearing plants that are not available today, but we still have a very large selection of delicious seed-bearing plants available to us. As nutritional research continues to uncover more healing properties and nutritional value of seed-bearing plants, we are coming to realize how vitally important it is to eat more of them!

THE GARDEN OF EDEN DIET
(PARTIAL LIST OF PRESENT-DAY VARIETIES)

GRAINS
AMARANTH, BARLEY, BROWN RICE, BUCKWHEAT, CORN, MILLET, OATS, QUINOA, RYE, SPELT, TEFF, WHEAT, WILD RICE

BEANS AND LEGUMES
ADZUKI BEANS, BLACK BEANS, BLACK-EYED PEAS, KIDNEY BEANS, LIMA BEANS, LENTILS, MUNG BEANS, NAVY BEANS, NORTHERN BEANS, PEANUTS, PINTO BEANS, SNAP PEAS, SOYBEANS, STRING BEANS, SWEET PEAS, WAX BEANS

NUTS
ALMONDS, BRAZIL NUTS, CASHEWS, PECANS, PINON, WALNUTS, FILBERTS

SEEDS
CHIA, FENNEL, FLAX, POPPY, PUMPKIN, PYSLLIUM, SESAME, SUNFLOWER

VEGETABLES
ARTICHOKES, ASPARAGUS, BEETS, BROCCOLI, BRUSSEL SPROUTS, CABBAGE (CHINESE RED AND GREEN), CARROTS, CAULIFLOWER, CELERY, COLLARDS, CUCUMBER, ENDIVE, GARLIC, JERUSALEM ARTICHOKES, KALE, KOHLRABI, LEEKS, LETTUCE (BIB, HEAD, RED LEAF, ROMAINE), MUSHROOMS, OKRA, ONIONS (RED, WHITE, YELLOW, SCALLION), PARSLEY, PARSNIPS, PEPPERS (GREEN, HOT, RED, YELLOW), POTATOES (IRISH, RED, SWEET, AND YAM), RHUBARB, RUTABAGA, SPINACH, SQUASH (ACORN, BUTTERNUT, HUBBARD, PUMPKIN, SPAGHETTI, YELLOW, ZUCCHINI), TOMATOES, TURNIPS, WATERCREST
(TO NAME A FEW)

FRUITS
APPLES (ALL VARIETIES), AVOCADO, APRICOTS,

BANANAS, BERRIES (BLUE, BLACK, CRANBERRIES, RASPBERRIES), CHERRIES, CURRANTS, DATES, FIGS, GRAPEFRUIT, GRAPES (CONCORD, GREEN, RED,WHITE), KIWI, LEMONS, MANGOS, MELONS (CANTALOUPE, CASABA, HONEYDEW, WATER-MELON), ORANGES, PAPAYAS, PEACHES, PERSIM-MONS, PINEAPPLES, PLANTAIN, PLUMS, POME-GRANATE, PRUNES, RAISINS, STRAWBERRIES, TANGERINES

HERBS AND SPICES

ALOE, BASIL, BAY LEAF, CARDAMON, CAYENNE, CINNAMON, CHILI POWDER, CORIANDER, CUMIN, CURRY, DILL, DONG QUAI, ECHINACEA, FRANKIN-CENSE, GARLIC, GINGER ROOT, GINSENG ROOT, GOLDENSEAL, MARJORAM, MUSTARD SEED, MYRRH, NUTMEG, ONIONS, OREGANO, PAPRIKA, PARSLEY, PINE BARK, ROSEMARY, SAFFRON, SAGE, SASSPARILLA, SASSAFRAS, TARRAGON, TUMERIC, THYME, WHITE WILLOW BARK, YUCCA
(TO NAME A FEW)

FRESH FOODS

Just as manna had to be eaten within a day or two or it would breed worms and stink (Exodus 16:20); all of God's foods: grains, beans, nuts, seeds, vegetables, and fruits are fresh and full of life-sustaining vitamins, miner-als and enzymes that need special care and proper stor-age. Man-made foods, because the life has been processed out of them, will stay on the shelves of your supermarket and in your cabinet almost indefinitely! God's foods, on the other hand, will spoil, rot, and decay if not eaten soon or stored properly - just like the manna!

Since the first man and woman had no oven to cook

their foods, unless God was the their chef (which is possible), they probably ate all their food uncooked or raw. Raw foods are easy to digest and none of the precious vitamins, minerals and enzymes are destroyed by the high temperatures of cooking. A health conscious person should eat **60 to 70 percent** of their foods raw or lightly steamed.

God's original and perfect diet of whole grains, protein-rich beans and legumes, raw nuts and seeds, fresh fruits and vegetables are the foundation of God's Nutrition Plan and should constitute **75 percent** or more of the total calories a health conscious person should eat each day. Our Creator knows better than any dietician, nutritionist or medical doctor what we need to eat to be well. After all, God did design our bodies and our digestive systems.

EXAMPLES

There are many examples in the Scriptures of godly people being grateful for God's provision of grains, seeds, nuts, fruits, and vegetables. Abraham, Daniel, Joseph, David, Moses, and many others knew the importance of the seed-bearing plants. They did not rebel against God's dietary recommendations by lusting after strange or exotic foods. Their faithfulness and odedience to follow the Creator's instructions with a thankful heart resulted in long and healthy lives. Even though some of the prophets and other Bible characters, including Jesus, occassionly ate clean meat and fish, seed-bearing plants remained the foundation of their diet and seed-bearing plants must be the foundation of our diet as well. Let us not complain about eating more grains and vegetables as the children of Israel did, but let us be thankful for these life-sustaining foods.

"Now these things became our examples, to the

intent that we should not lust after evil things as they lusted....Now all of these things happened to them as examples, and they were written for our instruction, on whom the ends of the ages have come."
(I Corinthians 10:6,11)

CHAPTER THREE

BEYOND THE GARDEN
(CLEAN AND UNCLEAN FOODS)

"You shall take with you seven each of every clean animal, a male and his female; two each of animals that are unclean, a male and his female."
(Genesis 7:2)

NOAH AND HIS FAMILY

The Lord saw that the wickedness and violence of man in the earth was great and **"that every intent of the thoughts of his heart was only evil continually." (Genesis 6:5)** The Lord decided to destroy both man and beast for He was grieved in His heart that He had made man on the earth. But one man, Noah, and his family found favor in the eyes of the Lord because **"Noah was a just man, perfect in his generations. Noah walked with God." (Genesis 6:9)**

After Noah built the ark, God gave him specific instructions concerning the animals that were to be brought into the ark (see Genesis 7:2 above). For the first time Scripture makes a distinction between animals - the clean and the unclean. How did Noah and his family **know** which animals were **clean** and which were **unclean**? God must have taught them! Whether the Lord taught them by bringing the clean and unclean animals in their

45

proper numbers onto the ark or whether Noah picked out the clean and unclean animals as they came to him is uncertain from the Scripture. But one fact is certain; after the waters subsided and Noah and his family left the ark, Noah sacrificed the <u>clean</u> animals and birds:

"Then Noah built an altar to the Lord, and took of every clean animal and of every clean bird, and offered burnt offerings on the altar."
(Genesis 8:20)

Noah understood which animals were clean and which were unclean, and he also knew that God **only** accepted the sacrifices of clean animals and birds. How did Noah know these important details? God instructed Noah about clean and unclean animals as Noah "walked with God".

After the great flood, God no longer limited man's diet to the "green herbs or plants". In addition to the original "garden diet" of grains, beans, nuts, seeds, fruits, and vegetables, which are considered clean and healthy by our Creator, God gave man permission to eat certain flesh foods.

"Every moving thing that lives shall be food for you. I have given you all things, even as the green herb."
(Genesis 9:3)

Would God give Noah permission to eat unclean animals, even though He would not accept them as sacrifices? Aren't the animals God calls clean for sacrifices, the same clean animals that He calls clean to eat in Leviticus 11 and Deuteronomy 14? Since Noah and his family were taught the law of clean and unclean (Genesis

7:2), they realized that eating **"all things"** meant that they could now eat the clean animals, birds and fish just as they could eat the clean grains, beans, nuts, seeds, fruits and vegetables. By the command of God, Noah and his family added to their vegetarian diet all the animals that the Lord considered to be **clean.** The Noahic Covenant (Genesis 9:9) established the eating of clean meats, excluding the blood (Genesis 9:4). God's permission to include only the clean animals, birds, and fish was later written down in great detail in the Mosaic Covenant.

AGES OF THE PATRIARCHS SHORTENED

Before the flood, the patriarches lived incredibly long lives eating a vegetarian diet of seed-bearing plants and trees; Adam-930 years, Seth-912 years, Enosh-905 years, Cainan-910 years, Mahalalel-895 years, Jared-962 years, Methuselah-969 years, Lamech-777 years, and Noah-950 years. Most of the inhabitants of earth, at the time of the great flood, were leading such self-indulgent, sinful and destructive livestyles that God decided to shorten mankind's lifespan:

"And the Lord said, 'My Spirit shall not strive with man forever, for he is indeed flesh; yet his days shall be one hundred and twenty years.' "

(Genesis 6: 3)

After the flood, with the introduction of animal foods, the average age of mankind decreased dramatically. Some Bible scholars suggest that the rapid decline in longevity was due to major environmental changes brought about by the flood. Although the likelihood of these climatic changes are very possible, this explanation is still a theory. What is a Biblical fact and not a theory, is that mankind began eating meat immediately after the flood and mankind's longevity took a drastic decline.

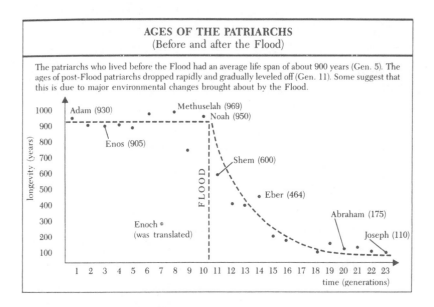

AGES OF THE PATRIARCHS
(Before and after the Flood)

The patriarchs who lived before the Flood had an average life span of about 900 years (Gen. 5). The ages of post-Flood patriarchs dropped rapidly and gradually leveled off (Gen. 11). Some suggest that this is due to major environmental changes brought about by the Flood.

NUTRITION GUIDANCE FOR ISRAEL

The Lord separated to Himself the children of Israel and gave them commandments and statutes full of wisdom and understanding. He wanted the nation of Israel to live a life that differed from the rest of the nations, even in the foods they ate. God first gave a husband and wife nutritional guidelines (Edenic Covenant), then a whole family (Noahic Covenant), and then an entire nation (Mosaic Covenant). Our heavenly Father wanted His children to live healthy, abundant lives for His purposes. That is why He told them what to eat. The whole grains and beans, raw nuts and seeds, and fresh fruits and vegetables remained through all the covenants as a clean and healthy foundation for **The Genesis Diet.** The seed-bearing plants, so vital to the health of all mankind, were a must for everyone; the flesh foods were optional.

YOU MAY EAT

In the garden diet, Genesis 1:29, God says "to you it **shall** be for food". The word **shall** is a **command** not a suggestion. The Lord is telling us that we have no option when it comes to eating grains, beans, nuts, seeds, fruits and vegetables—these seed-bearing plants are essential to our health. When the Lord outlines the instructions for eating clean flesh foods in Leviticus 11 and Deuteronomy 14, He says "you **may** eat" these meats. The word **may** is not a command, but rather gives us **permission** or the option to eat animal foods. We must eat (**shall eat**) the vegetables, but when it comes to meat, poultry, or fish, the Lord gives us the choice (**may eat**).

EDIBLE OR CLEAN ANIMALS

Clean and unclean foods are not related to whether something has been washed or not. The word **clean** means **edible**, and the word **unclean** means **not edible.** The Ultimate Nutritionist, Creator of all things tells us:

"These are the animals which you may eat: the ox, the sheep, the goat, the deer, the gazelle, the antelope....and you may eat every animal with cloven hooves, having the hoof split into two parts, and that chews the cud, among the animals."

(Deuteronomy 14:4-6)

How does a person tell what animals are edible? By observing two important facts about the animal—does it have **divided hooves and does it chew its cud (Deuteronomy 14:6, Leviticus 11:3)** The only animals that have both divided hooves **and** chew their cud are the **vegetarian animals** or herbivores (plant eaters). Herbivores are the healthiest of all the beast of the field because they don't eat the flesh of animals thereby avoiding the many diseases, parasites, and worms that are in the flesh and blood of those animals. Not only are vegetarian animals **free** of most diseases and parasites associated with the eating of flesh foods, but their long digestive tract which is six to twelve times the length of their bodies insures that they will completely process and eliminate any unfavorable toxins and poisons. **An edible or clean animal according to the Bible is defined by what it eats and the cleanliness of its digestive tract!** Besides the edible animals mentioned above we can add the cow and the buffalo because they also have divided hooves and chew their cud.

UNCLEAN ANIMALS

God identifies animals that are not edible as unclean animals, that is to say, not fit for human consumption. Unclean animals may exhibit one or the other criteria needed for them to be edible but **not both**; therefore, God commands "you **shall not** eat" these!

"Nevertheless, of those that chew the cud or have cloven hooves, you shall not eat, such as these: the camel, the hare, and the rock hyrax; for they chew the cud but do not have cloven hooves; they are unclean to you. Also the swine is unclean for you,

because it has cloven hooves , yet does not chew the cud; you shall not eat their flesh or touch their dead carcasses."

(Deuteronomy 14:7-8)

The **unedible** or **unclean** animals include: the camel (horses are included in this class), the hare or rabbit and the rock badger (this class includes all rodents, rats, squirrels, and mice) and the swine (this class includes bears, monkeys, bacon, ham, and sausage). **The entire group of unclean animals are called omnivores.** Omnivores eat both vegetation and animal foods. Omnivores will, by their very biological nature, eat anything! Their digestive tracts are much shorter than the herbivores because the decaying flesh and by-products are potentially toxic and must be removed from their body quickly.

THE SWINE

Obviously, the indiscriminate eating patterns of omnivores like pigs make them **disease carriers**. Pigs are known to carry up to 200 diseases and 18 different parasites and worms, including the deadly worm called trichinella spiralis. This worm is commonly called trichinosis and there is no known cure for these spiral worms. The trichinae worms are so small and transparent that only trained inspectors using high-powered microscopes can detect their existence. Trichinosis can cripple or even kill anyone that eats as little as a forkful of contaminated food! Trichinosis can mimic other diseases such as arthritis, rheumatism, or typhoid fever.

Pigs have more incidences of arthritis than any other known animals in the world. Arthritis may be a virus or a parasite that is transmitted from pigs to humans as a direct result of eating the flesh and blood of hogs or pigs. Perhaps many other diseases are misdiagnosed and their real cause is roundworm, gullet worms, hookworms, thorn-headed worms, trichina worms, stomach worms, nodular worms, tapeworms, as well as many other parasites found in the flesh of the **unclean** swine. A person may be committing slow suicide when they eat bacon, ham, sausage, or pork chops.

Even hog farmers who insist that corn fed hogs are safe won't give you a guarantee that their indoor hogs haven't eaten any rats, mice, fecal waste, or maggots within the past few days. The metal doorknobs in pig nurseries become corroded after a year or so due to the gases produced by the pigs urine and feces. The same gases and pig dander that eat away metal doorknobs are harming the respiratory tracts of hog farmers. Their unusually high incidences of respiratory ailments, from coughing and sniffles to lung scarring and pneumonia can no longer be attributed to weather and allergies alone. The hog waste spills from hog farms are contaminating our land, our rivers, and our water supply. Pork should be considered a homotoxin (human poison) and the probable cause of many common sicknesses and degenerative diseases.

The Great Physician, the Creator of all life, admonishes us to separate the clean animals from the unclean for physical health and well being. Many faithful church people who would never defile God's temple with cigarettes, even though smoking is not mentioned in the Bible, continue to ingest bacon, ham and pork chops which are disease-carrying, parasite-infested unclean foods which God commands His children not to eat! It would be futile and absurd to ask God to bless the smoking of cigarettes, yet we pray that He bless a pork chop on our dinner plate! Can we expect our Creator to disregard His word to us so we can indulge our appetites?

JESUS AND THE HOGS

Let us also remember the animals Jesus permitted the legion of demons to enter.

"And the demons begged Him saying, 'Send us to the swine, that we may enter them.' And Jesus gave them permission. Then the unclean spirits went out and entered the swine (there were about two thousand); and the herd ran violently down the steep place into the sea, and drowned in the sea."

(Mark 5:12-13)

Our loving Messiah, Jesus, came to destroy the works of the devil, yet He gave the demons permission to kill all those pigs! Jesus allowed unclean spirits to enter unclean animals.

EDIBLE OR CLEAN FISH

"These you may eat of all that are in the waters: you may eat all that have fins and scales."

(Deuteronomy 14:9)

The waters mentioned in this passage include the rivers, seas, and oceans (Leviticus 11:9). The clean or edible fish having **both** fins and scales are: bass, cod, flounder, grouper, haddock, halibut, herring, mackerel, orange roughy, perch, sole, salmon, red snapper, trout, tuna, and any other fresh or salt water fin and scale fish.

   Although fish contain a high percentage of cholesterol (see chart below), their total fat content is about half of that found in animal meats. The fats (5%-40%) that fin and scale fish contain are called omega-3 fatty acids. The fin and scale fish are especially rich in two of these omega-3 fatty acids:
   1. Dorosahexaenoic Acid (DHA)
   2. Eicosapentaeonic Acid (EPA)
   Scientific evidence suggests omega-3 fatty acids can decrease the risk of coronary heart disease and cancer. In the past, scientists believed all cholesterol was capable of clogging the arteries, but research now demonstrates that there is good cholesterol and bad cholesterol. The bad cholesterol or LDL (low density lipaproteins) is that part of the total cholesterol that contributes to heart disease and strokes. The good cholesterol, on the other hand, called HDL (high density lipaproteins), actually attaches itself to bad cholesterol in the arteries and carries it back to the liver for cleansing. Although fin and scale fish are high in cholesterol, the majority of the cholesterol is the good kind. This is not a fish story, it's true!

Fish	Measure	Calories	Protein (g)	Total Fat (g)	Cholesterol (mg)
Bass	1 lb	472	85.7	9.5	0
Cod	1 lb	354	9.8	3.31	227
Haddock	1 lb	358	83.0	2.99	272
Halibut	1 lb	454	94.8	4.98	227
Herring	1 lb	798	78.5	28.1	386
Mackeral	1 lb	566	86.2	44.4	431
Perch	1 lb	451	86.2	11.3	0
Salmon	1 lb	984	102	60.8	272
Snapper	1 lb	422	89.8	5.44	0
Trout	1 lb	885	97.5	51.7	249

*lb = pounds, (g) = grams, (mg) = milligrams
Composition of Foods, U.S. Agriculture Handbook No. 8

Meat	Measure	Calories	Protein (g)	Total Fat (g)	Cholesterol (mg)
Chuck Roast	1 lb	905	78.8	75	270
Club Steak	1 lb	1443	58.9	132	261
Ground Beef	1 lb	1216	81.2	96.2	307
Sirloin Steak	1 lb	1316	71.0	112.0	261
T-Bone Steak	1 lb	1596	59.0	168.0	261
Lamb Chop	1 lb	1146	63.7	97.0	270
Lamb Leg	1 lb	845	67.7	61.7	265
Pork Chop	1 lb	1065	61.0	89.0	260
Bacon	1 lb	3016	38.1	314	999
Ham	1 lb	1535	66.7	138	318
Veal Cutlet	1 lb	681	72.3	41	254
Chicken Breast	1 lb	394	74.5	18	239
Chicken Leg	1 lb	313	51.2	30.7	239
Turkey (light)	1 lb	798	149	37.6	458

*lb † pounds, (g) = grams, (mg) = milligrams
Composition of Foods, U.S. Agriculture Handbook No. 8

JESUS ATE CLEAN FISH

Jesus muliplied the two fish in one of His greatest miracles, ate fish Himself (Luke 24:42-43), and cooked a breakfast of fish for His disciples (John 21:9-12). All the clean fish eaten in Bible times were freshly caught and eaten; none were frozen or canned.

WARNING ON FISH

Fish is one of the most perishable of all foods. **Bacteria is the main cause** in the spoilage process, although natural enzymes and oxygen in the air also contribute to the break down of the flesh of dead fish. When ocean fish begin to spoil, they produce a compound called "trimethylamine" which causes the "fishy" odor. **Fresh fish have no odor**. Time and temperature are common enemies of freshness and flavor. Bacteria multiply rapidly when fish are out of the water too long or are stored at temperatures that are too high. If you choose to eat

fish remember these 3 important points:
>   1. Eat very fresh fish (no frozen or fresh frozen),
>   2. Choose only the clean varieties
>   3. Never eat them raw or undercooked.

Today, even God's clean fish must swim in rivers and oceans which are dumping grounds for potentially harmful chemicals like synthetic liquids (PCBs), mercury, lead, and a long list of pesticides that have been used on land. Once in the water, these substances make their way into sediments at the bottom and into aquatic plants and animals at the base of the food chain. Little fish eat plants and little animals, bigger fish eat little fish, and so on up the food chain. Fish also absorb substances directly from the water that passes over their gills.

UNCLEAN FISH

"And whatever does not have fins and scales you shall not eat; it is unclean for you."

(Deuteronomy 14:10)

Alright , we don't eat crocodiles, snakes, or intelligent dolphins. But the list of unclean fish includes some of our favorite main courses: shark (no scales), swordfish (no scales), catfish (no scales), and those delicacies that have neither fins or scales - shrimp, lobster, crab, clams, scallops, and snails. God tells us that these unclean fish are an **abomination** to us, four consecutive times in three verses:

"But all that are in the seas or in the rivers that do not have fins and scales, all that move in the water or any living thing which is in the water, they

are an abomination to you. They shall be an abomination to you; you shall not eat their flesh, but you shall regard their carcasses as an abomination. Whatever in the water does not have fins and scales— that shall be an abomination to you."
(*Leviticus 11:10-12*)

Nowhere else in Scripture does the Lord repeat, four consecutive times, such a stern warning. Does God think we are deaf or blind or does He foresee our lustfulness for these "scavenger" fish. The word **abomination** is defined as "anything that arouses strong disgust; a revolting thing; a loathing, hatred of, strong dislike for, or detestable." God puts great emphasis on how detestable shellfish are to eat. These scavenger fish are cesspools of filth, containing high levels of cholesterol, mercury, disease, worms, chemicals, and parasites. They are as unhealthy for us to eat as swine, rats, or cockroaches! God knew how perverted our taste buds would become and speaks to us:

"I have stretched out My hands all day long to a rebellious people, who walk in a way that is not good, according to their own thoughts;..... Who eat swine's flesh, and the broth of abominable things is in their vessel."
(*Isaiah 65:2-4*)

There's that word **abominable** again! Could our Lord be referring to clam chowder in those vessels? Oysters, clams, and mussels are immobile "filter feeders" shellfish that sit in one spot in shallow areas near population centers and pump water through their bodies to soak up nutrients. Along with their lunch, they often accumulate a dangerous dose of bacteria and viruses from human sewage! Can you imagine a person slurping down whole raw oysters, clams, or mussels-including the entire digestive tract! They do! Raw oysters, clams, and other such shellfish may also harbor hepatitis. As if that weren't enough to keep you away from these shellfish, deadly nerve toxins called "red tides" can strike eaters of even well-cooked shellfish. The symptoms range from paralysis to memory loss. The problem with all shellfish stems from their very nature — God created these "cockroaches of the ocean" to clean up the waters, but not to be eaten.

CLEAN AND UNCLEAN BIRDS

The Lord tells us we may eat the clean birds in **Deuteronomy 14:11** and then proceeds to give us a long list of birds we may not eat in **Deuteronomy 14:12-18** and **Leviticus 11:13-19** The unedible birds include the eagle, vulture, buzzard, falcon, raven, ostrich, owl, sea gull, hawk, stork, and bat (YUM!). All of these unclean "birds of prey" eat the flesh of man and beast, taking into their feathery bodies every disease and parasite of the animals they devour. Oh, what wisdom and common sense our Creator gives to those who will receive it. **The edible birds would include:**

1. chicken 2. turkey 3. duck 4. quail
5. cornish hen.

WARNING ON POULTRY

The director of the microbiology division of the United States Food and Drug Adminstration's Center for Food

Safety and Applied Nutrition, Joseph M. Madden, Ph.D., estimates that as much as 70% of chicken is laced with bacteria such as salmonella and campylobactor, up from estimates of 37% in the 1970's. In processing plants, the slaughtered chickens containing some residual feces are dumped into a **"chiller"** (a huge refrigerated bath). The chiller is basically toilet water and if the birds aren't haboring salmonella, campylobactor, E. coli, and other bad bugs when they go into the chiller, they probably are when they come out!

Most of what contaminates poultry are weak bacteria that are easily destroyed by enough heat; thoroughly cooked chicken is more likely to be bacteria-free. Grilling results in many cases of food poisoning because chicken grilled or barbecued on too high a flame may be charred on the outside and remain pink on the inside, possibly harboring harmful bacteria. Here are a few rules that will help prevent infection from poultry:

1. Wash your hands and utensils in hot soapy water after handling raw poultry or meat.

2. Use machine-washable plastic or marble cutting boards, never wood which has crevices that can hide bacteria for months.

3. Buy grain fed, antibiotic, chemical-free chickens and turkeys. Call your local health food store for a recommendation on where to buy "organic" poultry.

4. Drain the blood by soaking in salt water or call a synagogue to find out where to buy kosher (blood-drained) poultry.

CLEAN AND UNCLEAN WINGED INSECTS

Most civilized people don't eat flying insects and God does tell us in **Leviticus 11:21** not to eat **"of every flying**

insect that creeps on all fours: those which have jointed legs above their feet with which to leap on the earth." However, God does list a few edible insects:

"These you may eat: the locust after its kind, the destroying locust after its kind, the cricket after its kind, and the grasshopper after its kind"

(Leviticus 11:22)

Don't those sound yummy? Anyone for grasshopper stew or a cricket sandwich? Yet as revolting as these insects are to "civilized" folk, God would rather us eat locust or grasshoppers than ham, bacon, pork chops, shrimp, lobster, or crab legs!

HAVE YOU FOUND HONEY?

Honey is a product of **winged insects**. Many people believe honey is much healthier than refined sugar. After all, honey is a natural product of bees and white sugar is man-made and processed sugar. What most people don't realize is that **honey is twice as sweet as sugar** and it **sticks to your teeth better than sugar!**

Honey, sometimes referred to as the "nectar of the gods", doesn't have much more nutritional value than processed white sugar! The Bible warns us:

"It is not good to eat much honey; . . ."

(Proverbs 25:27)

Why isn't it good to eat much honey? Two good reasons have already been mentioned and the Bible adds yet another good reason in **Proverbs 25:16**.

"Have you found honey? Eat only as much as you need, Lest you be filled with it and vomit."

	SUGAR 1 Tablespoon	HONEY 1 Tablespoon	1 Tablespoon Honey's contribution to daily need of adult man.
Protein (g)	0	tr	◁ 1/100
Calcium (mg)	0	1	◁ 1/100
Iron (mg)	tr	0.1	◁ 1/100
Vitamin A (IU)	0	0	0
Thiamin (mg)	0	tr	◁ 1/100
Riboflavin (mg)	0	0.01	◁ 1/100
Niacin (mg)	0	0.1	◁ 1/100
Vitamin (mg)	0	tr	◁ 1/100

vs.

At first glance, honey looks more nutritious than sugar but when compared to a person's nutrient needs, neither contributes anything to speak of. Calculations are from Appendix H, Items 541 and 550, and the U.S. RDA. Nutrition Concepts and Controversies (Hamilton & Whitney)

mg = milligrams
g = grams
tr = trace
◁ = less than
IU = International Units

Because honey is highly concentrated and, like sugar, it is acid-forming to the digestive system, perhaps that is why the Bible recommends eating only a small amount of honey at a time. Although small amounts of honey are better than sugar, the natural sugars found in grains, starchy vegetables like carrots and potatoes, and fresh or dried fruits are the best alternatives. When you are baking, natural sweetners derived from grains such as brown rice syrup, barley malt syrup, and rice bran syrup or fruit juice concentrates, apple juice concentrate syrup, as well as maple syrup and honey in small amounts are excellent substitutes for sugar.

DON'T EAT CREEPY THINGS

In some parts of the world lizards are a delicacy, but for most of us, God's list of unedible creeping things doesn't bring tears to our eyes:

"These also shall be unclean to you among the creeping things that creep on the earth: the mole, the mouse, and the large lizard after its kind; the gecko, the monitor lizard, the sand reptile, the sand lizard, and the chameleon...And every creeping thing that creeps on the earth shall be an abomination. It shall not be eaten."
(Leviticus 11:29-30 ,41)

GOD'S EDIBLE FLESH FOODS

CLEAN MEATS
ANTELOPE, BUFFALO, CATTLE, DEER, GOAT, OXEN, SHEEP AND ANY OTHER ANIMAL WITH DIVIDED HOOVES AND CHEWS THE CUD

CLEAN FISH
BASS, COD, GROUPER, HADDOCK, HALIBUT, HERRING, MACKEREL, ORANGE ROUGHY, PERCH, SALMON, SNAPPER, TROUT AND ANY OTHER FIN AND SCALE FISH

CLEAN BIRDS
CHICKEN, CORNISH HEN, DUCK, QUAIL, TURKEY AND ANY OTHER NON-FLESH-EATING BIRD

WARNING ABOUT FLESH FOODS

Even though God chose the "healthiest" animals, birds, and fish for us to eat, we must not forget that flesh foods today are injected with growth hormones and antibiotics, live in polluted environments, and contain many strains of unhealthy bacteria and undetected viral infections. All flesh products are high in cholesterol and saturated fats. We must use Godly wisdom in selecting not only the clean or edible flesh foods but also in selecting naturally fed and raised, chemically-free animal foods as well.

The relaxation of federal regulations over the past twelve years has permitted farmers to raise animals in dangerously crowded conditions and meat packers to speed up processing lines. Unfortunately, these practices can pollute poultry and beef with fecal bacteria such as salmonella, campylobacter, E. coli, and clostridium—some of which are resistant to antibiotics. **According to the U.S. Centers for Disease Control, every year millions of Americans become sick from disease-causing bacteria or viruses in poultry, fish, and red meat.** One reason there hasn't been public outcry about this is that most of these millions of Americans only suffer from symptoms of diarrhea for a day or two, don't see a doctor, and blame their symptoms on stomach flu or even stress.

Ironically, as more and more people substitute poultry and fish for beef in an attempt to lower cholesterol and total fats from their diets, an increasing percentage of food-borne illnesses are being noted. The safest thing is to assume that all meat

63

is contaminated with disease-causing organisms. Many dangers exist in eating these foods carelessly and without restraint.

God insists in His word that all edible or clean animals, fish, and birds be freshly killed, the blood drained (fish excluded), the fat removed, and the flesh be well-cooked. Perhaps we should follow the instructions God gave to the children of Israel in Exodus 12:9-10 when cooking flesh foods and throw away any leftovers as well.

"Do not eat it raw, nor boiled at all with water, but roasted in fire .... You shall let none of it remain until morning ...."
(Exodus 12:9-10)

EAT NO BLOOD

A kosher or clean animal is slaughtered by cutting the throat with a very sharp knife and the blood is drained out of the animal. The words "pour out its blood" (Leviticus 17:13), and "you shall pour it (blood) on the earth like water" (Deuteronomy 12:24) refers to the proper slaughter of clean animals. Today we eat animals that have been killed by a "death blow" or a plastic bullet shot into their head and then the blood is drained. However, much of the blood enters the tissues and muscle of the animal when it is killed in this manner. God commands us not to eat the blood of clean animals:

"Only be sure that you do not eat the blood, for the blood is the life; you may not eat the life with the meat. You shall not eat it; you shall pour it on the

earth like water. You shall not eat it, that it may go well with you and your children after you, when you do what is right in the sight of the Lord. (Deuteronomy 12:23-25)

Since the life of the animal is in the blood, **"For the life of the flesh is in the blood" (Leviticus 17:11),** the opposite is also true. Death is in the blood. The blood absorbs what is in the stomach and circulates these products, good or bad, to the rest of the body. Most diseases of both man and animal find their way into the blood stream and the blood spreads the diseased cells to other locations within the body. If a mortician, otherwise known as an "undertaker", doesn't drain the blood out of a corpse soon after death, the body will decay very rapidly. Blood not drained out of an animal will flood that carcus with deadly putrefaction and disease. The Lord knew this fact and therefore instructed us to drain the blood.

Drinking blood is out, of course, as well as blood pudding and blood sausage. What about the blood contained in the beef, lamb, veal, chicken, and turkey we buy? Rare steaks and roasts are obvious sources of blood, and how we love those "tasty juices". Even well-cooked meats contain **delectable**, or is that **detestable**, juices full of the animal's blood. How do we get rid of the blood of clean animals we desire to eat? **The only way to properly slaughter and drain the blood is the kosher method.** All other methods are equivalent to strangulation. The penalty for eating the blood is pain, sickness, disease, and even death.

BE HOLY

God concludes the chapter in Leviticus on clean and unclean flesh foods in a very surprising way. To most of us, food has nothing to do with holiness, yet God closes the "food" chapter with this:

"For I am the Lord your God. You shall therefore sanctify yourselves, and you shall be holy; for I am holy."

(Leviticus 11:44)

God wants us to be holy, because He is holy. The word **holy** is defined as **"belonging to God; set apart for God's service; coming from God."** We belong to God. God is calling us to live a life set apart to Him because we belong to Him. We are called to holy living. Food is only one of many aspects of living where God has given us specific instructions for holy living. The world worships idols and food is one of those idols:

"And what agreement has the temple of God with idols? For you are the temple of the living God. ....Therefore, Come out from among them and be separate, says the Lord. Do not touch what is unclean, and I will receive you."

(2 Corinthians 6:16-17)

The Lord is calling us out of unholy living and to separate ourselves to His standard of holiness. **When we choose to honor the things that God honors, we set ourselves apart for His purposes to be fully realized in our lives.** Since we are triune beings, spirit, soul, and body, each area must be set apart or sanctified to God for

His use. When we sanctify or choose not to participate in what the Lord calls filthiness or unclean, we are perfecting holiness:

"Therefore, having these promises, beloved, let us cleanse ourselves from all filthiness of the flesh and spirit, perfecting holiness in the fear of the Lord."
(2 Corinthians 7:10)

We are to present our body each day as a living sacrifice, holy and acceptable to God which is our reasonable service (Romans 12:1) until the day of Messiah's return:

"Now may the God of peace Himself sanctify you completely; and may your whole spirit, soul, and body be preserved blameless at the coming of our Lord Jesus Christ. He who calls you is faithful and who also will do it."
(I Thessalonians 5:23)

Our loving God commands us in **Leviticus 11:47 "to distinguish between the unclean and the clean, and between the animal that may be eaten and the animal that may not be eaten."** Since God is holy, choosing to obey His commandments is choosing holiness. One of the ways God shows His love for us is through His commandments and one of the ways we demonstrate our love for Him is by keeping His commandments. The Scriptures tell us:

"For this is the love of God, that we keep His commandments. And His commandments are not burdensome." (I John 5:3)

CHAPTER FOUR

ALL THE FAT IS THE LORD'S
(GIVE IT TO HIM)

"....and the priest shall burn them on the altar as food, an offering made by fire for a sweet aroma; all of the fat is the Lord's"
(Leviticus 3:16)

The burning of animal fat is a **"sweet aroma"** for anyone who has smelled a sizzling steak as it cooks over mesquite wood, or barbecued ribs on an outdoor grill, or bacon crackling in a frying pan. The aroma of burning fat draws millions to buy hamburgers and french fries at their favorite fast food restaurant. Let us not forget the tantalizing aroma of fresh hot donuts that have been boiled in oil. **But to the Lord there is only one purpose for animal fat - as an offering to be burned on an altar as a sweet aroma.** The Lord says that all animal fat belongs to Him and is not to be eaten:

"This shall be a perpetual statute throughout your generations in all your dwellings: you shall eat neither fat nor blood."
(Leviticus 3:17)

BAD FATS

Moses and the children of Israel may not have comprehended or appreciated the health risks associated with
animal fats because they did not have the advantage of
the American Heart Association warning them through
the media as we do. But today, most everyone has heard
something about the dangers of eating animal fat. Animal fat is a hard, **saturated fat**, high in cholesterol, and
one of the main culprits in the development of arterioscle-
rosis, heart disease, strokes, diabetes, various forms of
cancer and obesity. About 43% of the calories consumed
by the average American comes from animal fats. The
American people devour large amounts of meats, poultry,
milk, and cheese, yet the Lord says:

".....You shall not eat any fat
of ox or sheep or goat."
(Leviticus 7:23)

The Biblical references forbidding the eating of animal
fat can be well understood by believers and non-believers
alike in this modern era of nutritional information. High
cholesterol and triglyceride levels are linked in countless
scientific studies to increased risks of coronary heart
disease, high blood pressure, hypertension, and arterio-
sclerosis. The popularity of fast food chains across
America accounts for over 15 billion dollars in revenues
each year. Burgers, fries, donuts, and shakes are high in
calories with more than 50% of those calories coming from
saturated fat. The American Cancer Society and the
National Cancer Institute warn people of the dangers of
excess animal fat, especially fried, rancid animal fat (free-
radicals) contributing to higher incidences of cancer.
Animal fats are the **"bad fats"** that the Lord told us not
to eat 3,500 years ago.

OVERWEIGHT OR OVERFAT

Animal fat, which is eaten in great abundance throughout America, is not only responsible for heart problems and cancer, but also for obesity. The over-consumption of high fat foods has created an epidemic of obesity in the U.S. with 2 out of every 5 Americans overweight. Weight loss clinics and weight loss products are a multi-billion dollar industry! We are overweight (40% of the American population) because we eat too much fat! Americans who consume 40% to 50% of their daily calories in fat are slowing their metabolism.

We are not only overweight due to fat accumulation, but we are accumulating fat to store toxins! The fat of an animal is where the poisons and toxins ingested by that animal are stored. Each gram of animal fat contains many toxins. The poisons in an animal's fat is transferred into the human body and stored in a human's fat cells. Overweight people are plagued with toxic weight gain from eating animal products. As a safety valve, these poisons are stored in the outer layers of the fat, rather than left to circulate in the blood and collect in the internal organs of the body. Severe calorie restricted diets not only starve God's temple, but quick weight loss diets release too many toxins from stored fat into the blood stream that can damage the liver, gallbladder, and kidneys.

LOSE WEIGHT GOD'S WAY

By restricting the unhealthy animal fats in our diets, which God commands, we can reduce the amount of total fat and toxins we consume. Reducing the total fat we eat will result in a slow, steady, and permanent weight loss. In my book, **Breaking the Fat Barrier,** a step-by-step plan for healthy weight loss is described. The premise of the book is that the determining factor in weight gain is not the total number of calories consumed each day, but the total amount of fat consumed! And the fat you want to trim away in your diet is animal fat. Reducing the health-destroying animal fats while consuming no more than 20% of the "good fats" each day stimulates metabolism and weight loss.

GOOD FATS

The "good fats" are the fats that come from the vegetable kingdom. Very few of these vegetable fats, with the exception of palm kernel oil and coconut, are saturated. On the contrary, vegetable oils are mostly **monounsaturated** or **polyunsaturated. All fats from the vegetable kingdom contain no cholesterol.** The clean fish also contain some polyunsaturated oils. As a rule, it is the saturated fats that tend to raise the level of bad cholesterol, or LDL (Low Density Lipoprotein), in the blood. On the other hand, the monounsaturated fats, such as olive oil, tend to lower the bad cholesterol by increasing the good cholesterol, or HDL (High Density Lipoprotein), which carries the bad cholesterol from the arteries back to the liver for processing.

Good fats can be subdivided into essential and nonessential fatty acids. The nonessential fatty acids can be manufactured by your body, essential fatty acids can not. The essential fatty acids (EFA) must be obtained through the foods you eat and vegetable fats are the very best source. Fish oils have essential fatty acids too, but fish also contains high levels of cholesterol. Essential fatty acids increase the metabolism of the body when they compose at least 12% to 15% of the total calories. **We need the "good fats" for an efficient metabolism!**

The following fats and oils chart reveals the superiority of vegetable fats over animal fats.

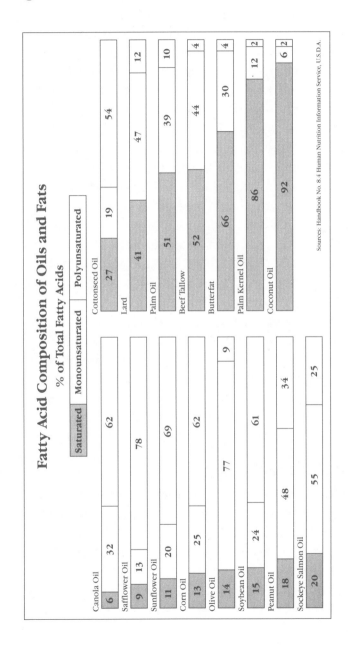

Fatty Acid Composition of Oils and Fats
% of Total Fatty Acids

	Saturated	Monounsaturated	Polyunsaturated
Canola Oil	6	62	32
Safflower Oil	9	13	78
Sunflower Oil	11	20	69
Corn Oil	13	25	62
Olive Oil	14	77	9
Soybean Oil	15	24	61
Peanut Oil	18	48	34
Sockeye Salmon Oil	20	55	25
Cottonseed Oil	27	19	54
Lard	41	47	12
Palm Oil	51	39	10
Beef Tallow	52	44	4
Butterfat	66	30	4
Palm Kernel Oil	86	12	2
Coconut Oil	92	6	2

Sources: Handbook No. 8.4 Human Nutrition Information Service, U.S.D.A.

OLIVE OIL

Olive oil is the finest and most nutritious of all the vegetable oils available. It is mentioned many times in the Bible and has been used since ancient times in religious practices where "anointing" of the sick (James 5:14) or priestly ordination was performed (Exodus 29:7, 30:24-25). Jesus and His disciples spent many hours of peace and prayer in an olive tree grove on the Mt. of Olives called Gethsemane (which means the oil press). Olive oil was used as fuel in the lamps of the Tabernacle (Exodus 27:20) and added to the unleaven bread offering in the Temple (Exodus 29:2). Olive oil is recommended by God!

There are many health benefits from including olive oil in your diet. Cultures who use large amounts of olive oil have lower rates of heart disease. Olive oil, being rich in essential fatty acids such as linoleic acid, provides substances necessary to build healthy glands and hormones as well as a good amount of vitamin E.

As you can see from the chart, olive oil has the highest percentage of monounsaturated fatty acids (77%). Monounsaturated fat is the least likely to become rancid. Rancid fats in the human body can lead to the development of free-radical formation which is carcinogenic or cancer-causing. Olive oil need not be refrigerated because of its high monounsaturated fat content; however, the polyunsaturated oils like safflower, corn, and peanut turn rancid very quickly and therefore must be refrigerated. Even exposure to light or heat can force the polyunsaturated oils to become rancid and therefore cooking with these oils at high temperatures is not recommended. Olive oil can be used for sauteing and stir-frying quite well.

When buying olive oil, a common question is: What does **"extra-virgin"** mean? After olives are picked, they are made into a paste which is spread on nylon matts. The matts are stacked and a hydraulic press sqeezes out the oil. The result is cold-pressed olive oil. (Only sesame and olive oil are pressed without heat or mechanical means.) The first pressing of the olive paste is called "extra-virgin", which not only tells the buyer that it is the first pressing, but also indicates the lowest amount of acid (less than 1%). **Approximately 40 olives are pressed to make one tablespoon of olive oil.**

The term **"pure olive oil"** could mean the second, third, or fourth pressing of the same olive paste and contain 3% to 5% acid. Extra-virgin olive oil is the most nutritious, but has the strongest taste. Extra-virgin olive oil should be packaged in amber-colored bottles or cans for longest protection and should be stored on a shelf in a cool, dark place. After purchasing olive oil, it should be consumed within a year's time.

Since ancient times, olive oil has been used by beautiful women around the world to feed and moisturize their skin and hair. Before retiring, rub two tablespoons of olive into hair. Comb or brush in thoroughly. Place a shower cap over head and leave on overnight. Shampoo in the morning. Hair is lusterous and healthy after feeding with this "olive oil bath".

Olive oil is truly a gift from God, promoted by God, and the best oil to add to salads, soups, cooked vegtables, stir-fried vegetables, and sauces. Fresh lemon juice can be added to olive oil to make a excellent natural salad dressing. An Italian legend says: "Once upon a time the trees decided to elect a king. After much deliberation, they elected the olive tree. The olive tree declined the honor, saying, 'The mission with which God has entrusted me, the well-being of mankind, is too important for me to distract myself with the duties of government.' "

THE ALMOND: KING OF THE NUTS

All raw, unsalted nuts are high in complete proteins, cholesterol-free fatty acids, fiber, vitamins, and minerals; however, the almond is, **"The King"**! The almond has the distinction of being the one and only alkaline-forming nut. All other nuts are acid forming. The almond's alkalinity makes it easier to digest especially for those with over-acid conditions such as ulcers. Almonds have generous amounts of calcium, magnesium, potassium, iron, vitamin B, vitamin C, vitamin E and protein. The United States Department of Agriculture has accepted the almond as **a meat alternative** in the National School Lunch Program.

COMPARISON: ALMOND vs. MILK (3½ oz.)				
NUTRIENT	ALMOND Raw Unsalted	*COW'S MILK 3.5% fat	COW'S MILK 3.7% fat	*SKIM MILK
CALCIUM	234mg	118mg	117mg	121mg
PROTEIN	18.6mg	3.5mg	3.5mg	3.6mg
FIBER	2.6mg	0	0	0
PHOSPHORUS	504mg	93mg	92mg	95mg
IRON	4.7mg	trace	trace	trace
POTASSIUM	773mg	144mg	140mg	145mg
THIAMINE	.24mg	.03mg	.03mg	.04mg
RIBOFLAVIN	.92mg	.17mg	.17mg	.18mg

*Pasteurized and raw
Source: U.S. Department of Agriculture Handbook #8.

Almonds, raw and unsalted, contain twice as much calcium as the same quantity of milk. Almonds are an excellent way of getting high quality calcium without using dairy products.

According to Scripture, almonds were given as gifts to kings and queens because of their reputation as a miracle food. Jacob tells his sons to take them as a gift to Joseph, in Egypt:

"And their father Israel said to them, 'Take some of the best fruits of the land in your vessels and carry down a present for the man....a little balm and a little honey, spices and myrrh, pistachio nuts and almonds.'"

(Genesis 43:11)

God's instructions for the design of the bowls in the Tabernacle, and later the Temple, were to resemble "almond blossoms" (Exodus 25:35). On the lampstand in the Holy Place, God commissioned artists to fashion almond branches and almond blossoms as ornamentation. (Exodus 25:34)

Aaron's rod, used to perform miracles, was none other than the branch of an almond tree:

"Now it came to pass on the next day that Moses went into the tabernacle of witness, and behold, the rod of Aaron, of the house of Levi, had sprouted and put forth buds, had produced blossoms and yielded ripe almonds."

(Numbers 17:8)

Aaron's miracle rod was ordered by the Lord to be placed in the Ark of the Covenant along with the stone tablets and the manna (Numbers 17:10, Hebrews 9:4). Other miracles God performed by using Aaron's rod include:

1. The rod became a serpent in front of Pharaoh (Exodus 7:9).
2. The rod swallowed up the sorcerers' serpents (Exodus 7:12).
3. The waters of Egypt turned to blood (Exodus 7:19).
4. Frogs came up and covered the land of Egypt (Exodus 8:5).
5. The dust of the earth became lice throughout Egypt (Exodus 8:16).

Almonds are an important part of the Genesis diet for problems of hunger control and weight loss and for their nutritional benefits. Eating six to eight almonds every few hours as a snack between main meals can help stabilize blood sugar and help prevent over-eating at meal times. They should always be eaten raw rather than roasted and salted. God has blessed us with the **"King of Nuts"**, one of the good fats for abundant health. Can you say "almond" to that!

UGLY FATS

Americans have attempted to cut down on their consumption of animal fats by eating more cholesterol-free vegetable oils. However, the overwhelming majority of these oils are in the form of **hardened vegetable fat!** Vegetable oil is naturally liquid at room temperature, so how do we end up with sticks of vegetable margarine? The processing of vegetable oil, called **hydrogenation,** forces hydrogen molecules into the structure of the polyunsaturated oil. Hydrogenation allows a manufacturer to use a cheap vegetable oil and **transform** it into a product that can compete with butter. The result of hydrogenation is the creation of a man-made fat called a **trans-fat.** These "new" trans-fatty acids resemble a saturated fat and can contribute to cardiovascular disease by inhibiting normal essential fatty acid metabolism and increasing the production of cholesterol.

FLESH POTS OF AMERICA

The flesh pots of Egypt to which the children of Israel wanted to return while in the wilderness, (Numbers11:4-21), would be equivalent to selected fast food restaurants Americans flock to today. Unfortunately, these modern day "flesh pots" serve foods that are 40% to 75% fat and most of those fats are meats, cheese, and other animal sources that pose a very high health risk.

Americans spend 50% of their food dollars eating out in fast food restaurants. Billions of dollars a year are wasted on these "fast foods" which are high in animal fat and low in nutritional content. This "deathstyle" of eating is making the United States one of the sickest nations in the world. The Lord speaks through the prophet Isaiah about purchasing foods that are lifeless and empty:

"Why do you spend money for what is not bread, And your wages for what does not satisfy? Listen diligently to Me, and eat what is good,...."
(Isaiah 55:2)

Following are the amounts of calories and fats in some of the favorite fast food restaurants:

NUTRITIONAL CONTENTS OF
SELECTED FAST FOODS

	Calories	Fat (Pats*)	Fat (Percent of calories)	Sodium (mg)
MCDONALD'S				
Hamburger	255	2.6	35	520
Chicken McNuggets	314	5.0	54	525
Filet-O-Fish	432	6.6	52	781
Big Mac	563	8.7	53	1,010
Sausage Biscuit	582	10.4	61	1,380
ROY ROGERS				
Plain Potato	211	0	0	65
Potato w/Oleo	274	1.9	24	161
Roast Beef Sandwich	317	2.7	29	785
Crescent Roll	287	4.7	56	547
Potato w/Broccoli 'n Cheese	376	4.8	43	523
Crescent Sandwich w/Sausage	449	7.7	59	1,289
Crescent Sandwich w/Ham	442	7.5	58	1,192
WENDY'S				
Pasta Salad (½ cup)	134	1.6	40	400
Chicken Sandwich on Wheat Bun	320	2.6	28	500
Taco Salad	390	4.8	40	1,100
Broccoli & Cheese Potato	500	6.6	45	430
Cheese Stuffed Potato	590	9.0	52	450
HARDEE'S				
Chef's Salad	272	4.2	53	517
Chicken Filet Sandwich	510	6.9	46	360
Shrimp Salad	362	7.7	72	941
Bacon Cheeseburger	686	11.1	55	1,074
ARBY'S				
Roasted Chicken Breast (no bun)	254	1.9	25	930
Broccoli & Cheese Potato	540	5.8	37	480
Mushroom & Cheese Potato	510	5.8	39	640
(Fried) Chicken Breast Sandwich	584	7.4	43	1,323
Sausage & Egg Croissant	530	9.3	59	745
LONG JOHN SILVER'S				
Baked Fish w/Sauce	151	0.5	12	361
Mixed Vegetables	54	0.5	33	570
Corn on the Cob	176	1.1	20	0
Coleslaw	182	4.0	74	367
Fish w/Batter (2 piece)	404	6.4	53	1,346
BURGER KING				
Veal Parmigiana	580	7.1	42	805
Bacon Double Cheeseburger	600	9.3	53	985
Specialty Chicken Sandwich	690	11.1	55	775
JACK IN THE BOX				
Shrimp Salad (no dressing)	115	0.3	8	460
Taco Salad	377	6.3	57	1,436
Chicken Supreme Sandwich	601	9.5	54	1,582
KENTUCKY FRIED CHICKEN				
Breast (Original Recipe)	199	3.1	53	558
Extra Crispy Dark Dinner**	765	14.2	63	1,480

*Pats-of-butter equivalent. A pat of butter contains 3.8 grams of fat.
**Includes drumstick, thigh, mashed potatoes, gravy, coleslaw, and roll.

We take our children into fast food restaurants to eat
foods which were once wholesome, but that man has
perverted into something that should no longer be classified as food. To **pervert** means to "to lead astray; misdi-
rect; corrupt; to misuse; to distort; twist." Certainly today
our taste buds have become perverted or corrupted, causing us to enjoy the taste of things that are harmful to our
health. Our Creator put the taste buds on the tongue!
With that in mind, the following verse takes on new
meaning!

"Death and life are in the power of the tongue,
And those who love it will eat its fruit."
(Proverbs 18:21)

Are we eating the foods that will produce the good
fruit of health and life in our bodies or are we partaking of
foods that will produce sickness and death in our mortal
bodies?

DAIRY PRODUCTS IN THE BIBLE

The Lord gave no milk or dairy products to Adam and
Eve when He designed the **garden diet** (Genesis 1:29),
nor do we find any mention of milk or dairy products in
the food chapters of Leviticus 11 or Deuteronomy 14 when
God gave Israel the dietary laws. Yet, the Lord described
the Promised Land as **"flowing with milk and honey"**.
This phrase is **symbolic** to describe the fertile, rich land
that would supply all of Israel's physical needs. By using
milk as an example, God was assuring the children of
Israel that the land He was taking them to was a place
that would nourish them just like breast milk nourishes a
newborn babe. In the same way, when God says in Genesis 45:18, **"you will eat the fat of the land,"** He does
not literally mean for us to eat fat. He is using symbolism

to describe the "choice produce" of the land.

Milk is also used symbolically in I Corinthians 3:2 where Paul is making an analogy between milk for babies and the elementary principles of Messiah for baby believers. This analogy is based upon a basic biological understanding that milk is for babies and solid food is for adults.

"I fed you with milk and not with solid food: for until now you were not able to receive it and even now you are not able."

(I Corinthians 3:2)

The theme of milk for the immature or baby believer is found in Isaiah 28:9-10, Hebrews 5:12, and elsewhere in the Scriptures. While our Creator designed female mammals to feed their young breast milk, no animal in nature continues drinking milk after it is weaned! These animals, including man, grow teeth which take them to the next stage of maturation - the eating of solid food. **If we examined the chemical constitution of each animal's milk, we would observe that the nutritional content of that milk is uniquely designed by our Creator for the specific needs of each animal specie.** For example, a cow's milk contains hormones which are secreted from the pituitary of the cow. These are powerful hormones designed to raise a calf from 90 pounds at birth to 1000 pounds at maturity two years later. By comparison, a human infant is 6-8 pounds at birth and reaches 100-200 pounds at maturity twenty-one years later! These cow hormones can unbalance the hormones of humans as well as contribute to large thighs and buttocks, all too common in American women.

THE KOSHER LAW AND MILK

An orthodox Jew does not eat milk products and meat together at the same meal because of the laws of kashrut (kosher). This kosher law is based on the verses in the Exodus 23:19 and Deuteronomy 14:21 that say:

"You shall not boil a young goat

in its mother's milk".

(Deuteronomy 14:21)

With all due respect to the rabbis of old, this verse does not command us to separate milk products from meat; therefore, the kosher law commanding two sets of dishes, one for dairy and the other for meat, is "a doctrine of men" rather than a commandment of God. Nowhere in the Bible does God tell us to separate the meat from the dairy. In fact, contrary to this rabbinic teaching, Abraham, the great father of faith, fed two angels and the Lord on their way to destroy Sodom and Gomorrah. This Scripture indicates that Abraham didn't practice the separation of milk and meat and apparently neither did the Lord since He ate what Abraham offered!

"So he (Abraham) took butter and milk and the calf

which he had prepared, and set it before them; and

he stood by them under the tree as they ate"

(Genesis 18:8)

ARE MILK PRODUCTS A HEALTH HAZARD?

There is great debate over the eating and drinking of dairy products. One side says dairy products cause mucus build-up, sinus congestion and infection, allergies, asthma, constipation and heart disease, while the other side, primarily the Dairy Council, claims "milk is nature's most perfect food." Cow's milk is nature's most perfect food for a calf, not for a human! We have the example of many healthy cultures around the world who use only small amounts of dairy products demonstrating that dairy products are not necessary to get enough calcium or to maintain optimum health. In fact, there is growing concern in the medical community that milk products can be harmful.

HOMOGENIZED MILK: CAUSE OF HEART DISEASE

Homogenized milk is milk that has been processed to breakup its fat content into very tiny particles so that they are evenly distributed. This prevents it from separating into cream as skim milk when it stands, as non-homogenized milk will do. The breakup of the fat into tiny particles allows xanthine oxidase (XO), an enzyme, to enter the blood stream and attack the heart and its arteries. This enzyme, XO, acts chemically to scar the artery wall and heart tissue. The body tries to repair the damage by manufacturing more cholesterol and depositing this protective fatty material (cholesterol) on the scars. If this process continues, the cholesterol begins to clog the arteries, causing heart disease.

MILK PRODUCTS: CAUSE OF ALLERGIES

Since each animal's milk is designed for the specific biological needs of the nursing young of that specie, **cow's milk has become the second leading cause of allergies among humans**. Humans seem to be allergic to the "casein", a type of protein, found in cow's milk. Human milk, on the other hand, contains lactoalbumin rather than casein. The allergic reactions to casein include the buildup of extra mucus in the lungs, throat, nose and sinuses as well as bloating, gas, and constipation. I call cheese "solidified mucus"!

MILK PRODUCTS: CAUSE OF DIGESTIVE PROBLEMS

Digestive difficulties from dairy products are caused because some people do not manufacture the digestive enzyme, **lactase**, produced by the pancreas to digest **lactose**, the sugar in milk. Perhaps that's why so many adults become bloated with gas from drinking milk and eating cheese. Since we are designed to drink human milk as babies, perhaps our bodies naturally stop producing the enzyme to digest milk sugar as adults. Milk was intended by God for infants whether animal or human, or else why would God have the breasts dry up after lactation? It seems that drinking cows milk as an adult is an unnatural nutritional act. Although not forbidden in the Bible, it is not recommended either.

IF YOU MUST.....

If you must drink milk, drink goat's milk rather than cow's milk. **Goat's milk is similar in nutritional composition to human milk** - cow's milk is not! The Scriptures refer to goats' milk for human food in Proverbs:

"You shall have enough goats' milk for your food, For the food of your household, And the nourishment of your maidservants."

(Proverbs 27:27)

For those mother's who are unable to breast feed, goat's milk diluted by one-third with distilled water would be far more natural and nutritious than man-made formulas. Goat's milk can also be used to make yogurt. Even cow's milk yogurt and kefir, which are curdled milk products, are easier to digest that straight milk or cheese. Curdled milk products contain a natural bacteria called acidophilus which acts as an enzyme to digest the lactose that is so difficult for adults to handle. The following Scripture suggests that during Bible times, they curdled cow's milk and drank the fresh, unhomogenized milk of goats and sheep.

"Curds from the cattle, and milk from the flock. . ."
(Deuteronomy 32:14)

CONCLUSION ON DAIRY

If milk is as important to nutritional health as TV ads and school books say it is, why didn't God command us to use it? Although the Bible speaks about milk, most of the verses refer to milk as the food of babies rather than adults. God designed baby mammals to live exclusively on their mother's milk until weaned to solid food. Since milk is the number two allergy-producing food in the United States and since many adults and young people experience digestive difficulties, sinus problems, constipation, and mucus buildup, not to mention that milk is an animal fat, it is best to use very little of it in your diet.

CHAPTER FIVE

DID GOD CHANGE
HIS MIND?
(GOD'S UNCHANGING WORD)

"For I am the Lord, I do not change."
(Malachi 3:6)

The Book of Malachi is the last book in the King James Version of the Old Testament. It is appropriate that before beginning the New Testament the Lord reminds us in Malachi 3:6 **"I do not change"** because some verses in the New Testament seem to contradict what He said earlier. Any Scriptures in the New Testament which seem to contradict Scriptures in the Old Testament are misunderstood and usually this misunderstanding can be traced to quoting verses out of their original context. **God's word is consistent from Genesis to Revelation.**

TEXT WITHOUT CONTEXT IS PRETEXT

When Yeshua (Jesus) was taken to the pinnacle of the temple in Jerusalem (Luke 4:9-12, Matthew 4:5-7), that old deceiver from the garden, satan, told Him to throw Himself down (jump) and quoted these verses from Psalm 91:11-12.

*"He shall give His angels charge concerning you,
and in their hands they shall bear you up, lest you
dash your foot against a stone."*

(Psalm 91:11-12)

Satan was attempting to persuade Jesus to jump off a building by insisting that God's word says His angels will protect Him! Here we have a classic example of satan quoting Scripture out of context in order to permit a behavior contrary to the Word and Will of God. Satan was tempting Jesus to doubt, deny, and defy the Word of God, just like he did with Adam and Eve in the garden!

Jesus knew the context of the verses satan was quoting to Him and therefore was not deceived. Jesus said to him:

*"It is written again, you shall not tempt
the Lord your God."*

(Deuteronomy 6:16)

The next verse in Deuteronomy after "You shall not tempt the Lord your God" is:

*"You shall diligently keep the commandments of
the Lord your God, His testimonies and
His statutes which He has commanded you."*

(Deuteronomy 6:17)

Any Scripture that sounds contrary to the commandments, testimonies, or statutes of God plays into the hands of the evil one and can cause great harm to the hearer. The Bible says, **"There is no God,"** not once but twice! A person could quote just this verse and make a case for people to be athiests. However, when we see this statement in its proper context we are correctly dividing the Word of God.

"The fool has said in his heart, 'There is no God.' "
(Psalm 14:1, 53:1)

Let us "rightly divide the the word of truth" by putting back into context a few New Testament Scriptures that have been used to convince some believers that God has changed His mind about clean and unclean foods.

ACTS 10: PETER'S VISION

"And a voice came to him, 'Rise , Peter; kill and eat.' But Peter said, 'Not so Lord! For I have never eaten anything common or unclean.' And a voice spoke to him again the second time, 'What I have cleansed you must not call common.' "
(Acts 10:13-15)

Many people point to Acts 10 as one of the places in the New Testament where God declares all foods to be clean. On the contrary, Acts chapter 10 isn't about food at all; it's about people. There are two stories in this chapter that are woven together into one glorious outcome: **taking the gospel to the Gentiles.** In order to understand the context of certain passages of Scripture in a chapter of the Bible, it is **often necessary to read the whole**

chapter! This is absolutely necessary for us if we want to understand what Acts 10:13-15 is really talking about.

START AT THE BEGINNING

The chapter begins with a description of a man named Cornelius, a centurion of the Italian Regiment living in Caesarea. Cornelius was a Gentile whose entire family feared the God of Abraham, Isaac, and Jacob (the God of the Jews). He prayed unceasingly and gave alms to the Jewish people. An angel of God spoke to Cornelius in a vision saying:

"Your prayers and alms have come up for a memorial before God. Now send men to Joppa, and send for Simon whose surname is Peter....He will tell you what you must do."

(Acts 10:4-6)

Cornelius sent two of his household servants and a loyal soldier to Joppa to speak to Peter:

"The next day, as they (servants of Cornelius) went on their journey and drew near the city, Peter went up on the house top to pray...."

(Acts 10:9)

This passage indicates that the servants from Cornelius, the Gentile, are somehow related to Peter's prayer. Peter became very hungry and while waiting for lunch to be served, fell into a trance:

"and saw Heaven opened and an object like a great sheet bound at four corners, descending to him and

let down to the earth. In it were all kinds of four-footed animals of the earth, wild beasts, creeping things, and birds of the air. And a voice came to him, 'Rise, Peter, kill and eat.' But Peter said 'Not so, Lord! For I have never eaten anything common or unclean!' And a voice spoke to him again the second time, 'What God has cleansed you must not call common.' This was done three times. And the object was taken up into Heaven again."

(Acts 10:11-16)

At this point in Acts 10, most people declare that Peter's vision nullifies the clean and unclean laws, but Peter was not so sure.

"Peter wondered within himself what this vision meant ."

(Acts 10:17)

Peter was definitely searching for the correct interpretation of this vision. **Would God want him to eat foods that are unhealthy and unclean to his body, which He commanded in His word not to eat?**

DREAMS AND VISIONS

It is important to mention that dreams in the Bible are generally **symbolic** rather than literal. For example, Pharaoh's dream in Genesis 41 of the seven fat cows and seven lean cows was symbolic and correctly interpreted by Joseph as seven plentiful years and seven years of famine. Another example is King Nebuchadnezzer's dream of a figure with a head of gold, chest and arms of silver, its belly and thighs of bronze, its legs of iron, and its feet partly iron and partly clay. This dream is correctly inter- preted by the prophet Daniel and the figure is explained as representing four successive kingdoms, each with less power and authority. Daniel also says something signifi- cant about dreams and visions in Daniel 2:28, **"But there is a God in heaven who reveals secrets, and He has made known . . .what will be in the latter days."** So Peter's vision is not literal but symbolic of something prophetic that was about to occur.

THE WHOLE TRUTH

Rather than stopping one third of the way through the chapter and insisting that God is nullifying His own nutritional principles, let's continue on to discover the true and vital message of this historic chapter. Let's review what we do know about Acts 10 thus far. First, men were sent to Peter from a Gentile named Cornelius on orders from an Angel of God (Acts 10:3). Secondly, Peter has a vision of unclean animals, unclean birds, and creeping things in which a voice tells him, "Rise Peter, kill and eat," and "What God has cleansed you must not call common." Thirdly, Peter's strong declaration to the Lord that he has never eat anything common or unclean is similiar to another very strong statement made by the prophet Ezekiel to the Lord regarding his faithfulness throughout his life to God's command to eat only clean foods:

"Ah, Lord God! Indeed I have never defiled myself from my youth till now; I have never eaten what

died of itself or was torn by beasts, nor has abominable flesh ever come into my mouth."
(Ezekiel 4:14)

While Peter was still thinking about the meaning of his vision, the Holy Spirit (The Spirit of Truth) merges these two seemingly different stories: 1. The visitation of an angel to Cornelius and 2. Peter's vision:

"While Peter thought about the vision, the Spirit of God said to him 'Behold, three men are seeking you. Arise, therefore, go down and go with them, doubting nothing; for I have sent them.' "
(Acts 10:19)

The Spirit of God, not merely an angel, commands Peter to go with these Gentile strangers whom God had sent to him. We begin to understand, as Peter began to understand, that these men are somehow related to his vision. Peter listens to the men's explanation that Cornelius is summoning him to Caesarea and the next day, the three men, Peter, and some believing Jewish brethern travel to the house of Cornelius in Caesarea (Acts 10:21-23). We can surmise that during the journey to Caesarea Peter had time to inquire of the Holy Spirit what these men and this vision had in common.

When Peter entered the house of Cornelius, the revelation which was to usher in **"The Time of the Gentiles"** was prophetically unfolding! Cornelius had invited his relatives and close friends to his home to hear Peter's words (Acts 10:24-27). The Apostle Peter finally understood the true significance of his vision as he spoke to those gathered in the house of Cornelius, the Gentile:

"You know how unlawful it is for a Jewish man to keep company with, or go to one of another nation. But God has shown me that I should not call any man common or unclean. Therefore, I came without objection as soon as I was sent for."
(Acts 10:28-29)

The Great Commission (Matthew 10:5-6, Luke 24:47) given by Jesus had been understood by the early church to mean to go into all the world and preach the gospel to the Jews who were dispersed among the Gentile nations (Matthew 10:5-6). Therefore, the gospel had only been preached to Jews even though several years had passed since Pentacost (the supernatural beginning of the New Covenant Church). Israel, God's chosen people, were commanded by God to be separated to Him, as a holy nation. All the other "nations" of the earth were "the Gentiles" and considered **unclean** because of their worship of "other gods". Jews were forbidden by God to intermarry with these "heathen nations" or assimilate into their cultures. According to Biblical prophecy Messiah would come to deliver Israel from the oppression of the Gentiles, sit on the throne of David in Jerusalem, and establish a world at peace with Israel.

How utterly taken off guard the brethern must have been to understand the mystery that was unfolding that day at Cornelius' house; the good news was not only to be preached to the Jews, but to the whole world! After hearing the explanation by Cornelius of the angelic visitation which instructed him to seek Peter out in Joppa (Acts 10:29-33), Peter had the full revelation:

"In truth I perceive that God shows no partiality. But <u>in every nation whoever</u> fears Him and works righteousness is accepted by Him. The word which God sent to the children of Israel, preaching peace through Jesus the Messiah———He is Lord of all!"
(Acts 10:34-36)

Now we can understand that the sheet on which there were unclean animals, birds, and creeping things, represented all the **unclean nations, the Gentiles,** to which the Jew should go and preach the gospel of the kingdom of God; for the blood of Jesus made a way for all men to become spiritually clean! The command in the vision to "Rise, Peter, kill and eat," was not to eat unclean things that are forbidden in Scriptures, but to enter the heathen nations and the houses of the Gentiles, in order to present the gospel to all those who would receive it.

THE PROPHETIC MEETING

This prophetic meeting of Peter, a Jew, with Cornelius and his Gentile relatives and friends was the beginning of the evangelism of the Gentiles. While Peter was still preaching the message of salvation to them:

"the Holy Spirit fell upon all those who heard the word. And those of the circumcision who believed were astonished, as many as came with Peter, because the gift of the Holy Spirit had been poured out on the Gentiles also."
(Acts 10:44-45)

In Acts chapter 11, when Peter visits the church in Jerusalem to tell them the amazing news of what had happened, some of the Jews there contended with him saying, "You went to uncircumcised men and ate with them!" But Peter explained the entire event to them from the beginning and:

"When they heard these things they became silent; and they glorified God, saying, 'Then God has also granted to the Gentiles repentance to life.' "
(Acts 11:18)

Acts chapter 10 marked the beginning of the "times of the Gentiles", not the end of clean and unclean foods. God was calling a remnant of Jewish believers to carry the good news of salvation into all the world:

"I, the Lord, have called you in righteousness, and will hold your hand; I will keep you and give you as a covenant to the people, as a light to the Gentiles."
(Isaiah 42:6)

"The Gentiles shall come to your light, and kings to the brightness of your rising."
(Isaiah 60:3)

In **"rightly dividing the Word of Truth"** (II Timothy 2:15), we can see that Peter's vision in Acts 10 was about people, not food, and the fulfillment of the the great commission to preach the gospel of salvation **"to the Jew first, and also to the Gentile"** (Romans 1:16).

"Go therefore and make disciples of all nations, baptizing them in the name of the Father and of the Son and of the Holy Spirit, teaching them to observe all things I have commanded you;"
(Matthew 28:19-20)

I TIMOTHY 4:4
(APPROVES SANCTIFIED FOOD)

"For every creature of God is good, and nothing is to be refused if it is received with thanksgiving;"
(I Timothy 4:4)

Another example of Scripture which is quoted out of context in order to approve the eating of unclean things, is **I Timothy, Chapter 4, verse 4.** Those who quote this verse insist that God is telling us to eat everything that He created. In order to interpret I Timothy 4:4 in this way, we must reject the clean and unclean laws of God, as well as endorse cannibalism! If we believe that God is telling us to eat poisonous snakes, rats, worms, spiders, and each other, then God would be contradicting His word and would not be the same yesterday, today, and forever (Hebrews 13:8)! The Word of God is consistent and carries a continuity and therefore, I Timothy 4:4 must have another interpretation which is consistent with the clean and unclean laws.

THE FOODS OF GOD

Paul, is the author of I Timothy and he is not making a distinction between creatures God created and those He did not create, for God created every creature. Every animal, every fish, every bird and every creeping thing is good because it was created by God. **But not everything God created was created to be eaten!**

FALSE DOCTRINE

We can avoid the "spirit of error" (I John 4:6) or false doctrine only by relying on the Scriptures as our final authority. The problem of false doctrine is the reason that Paul is discussing creatures we may eat in I Timothy chapter 4. In order to fully understand why Paul has brought up the issue of eating animals, I Timothy 4:4 must be read in its context, starting at the beginning of the chapter:

"Now the Spirit expressly says that in latter times some will depart from the faith, giving heed to deceiving spirits and doctrines of demons, speaking lies in hypocrisy, having their own conscience seared with a hot iron, forbidding to marry, and commanding to abstain from foods which God created to be received with thanksgiving by those who believe and know the truth."

(I Timothy 4:1-3)

Some people in the church of the first century were **"departing from the faith"** teaching false doctrines. These people were advocating celibacy (forbidding to marry) and vegetarianism (abstaining from certain foods or meats). This teaching or doctrine was forbidding activities that God desires His children to do. The Lord certainly ordained for us to marry and He created certain clean foods **"to be received with thanksgiving by those who believe and know the truth".** Those who believe and know what truth? The truth contained in the Scriptures which is our guide to correct doctrine. Being armed with the Sword of the Spirit, which is the Word of God (Ephesians 6:17), we are not likely to be **deceived** by a doctrine of demons. Deceiving spirits and doctrines of demons will contradict the Word of God and I Timothy 4:1-5 warns us not to believe a doctrine which tells us not to eat foods that God has permited for us to eat.

Now we understand that the purpose of the first part of I Timothy chapter 4 is to address a false teaching related to marriage and eating. If we believe and know the Word of God, such false doctrine would find no place in us. Paul finishes this discussion of the foods that the Lord created and sanctified (set apart) for us to eat by directing us back to His word:

"For it is sanctified by the Word of God

and prayer."

(I Timothy 4:5)

Paul is actually confirming to us in I Timothy 4:5 that we should eat only those creatures God has sanctified in His word. The **"it"** refers to those edible creatures that are "set apart" for us by God in Leviticus 11 and Deuteronomy 14. God's word is exact and precise so that the children of God may **"distinguish between the unclean and the clean, and between the animal that may be eaten and the animal that may not be eaten." (Leviticus 11:47)**

FOOD SANCTIFIED BY PRAYER

Since Jesus, a first century Hebrew, was eating only those foods that were clean, pure, and edible according to the Word of God; therefore, He never needed to ask God to bless His food. The food was already blessed by God. The only blessing required was to bless and thank <u>God</u> for His provision.

"When you have eaten and are full, then you shall bless the Lord your God for the good land which He has given you."
(Deuteronomy 8:10)

At the Lord's Supper, Yeshua(Jesus) took bread and blessed it. He probably spoke this ancient Hebrew prayer that is still used today at mealtimes:

"Blessed Art Thou, Oh Lord, our God, King of the Universe, who brings forth food from the earth."

There is an important difference between this traditional Hebrew blessing and the modern Christian dinner prayer that says something like, **"Bless this food to our bodies"**. God's word does not sanction the eating of a cobra cocktail, a rat roast, or a pig pie and all the well-meaning prayers said at the dinner table can not change the Word of God. On the contrary, our dinner prayers should bless God and be thankful to Him for setting apart (sanctifying) by His word, foods which have been created to keep us healthy.

THERE IS NOTHING UNCLEAN.... OR IS THERE?

*"I know and am conviced by the Lord Jesus
that there is nothing unclean of itself;
but to him who considers anything
to be unclean, to him it is unclean."
(Romans 14:14)*

WHAT IS CONSIDERED FOOD?

Today we consider almost anything **"food"**; from candy bars to frozen microwave dinners; from popcorn to donuts. The closest we come to labeling a substance **"unclean"** is to call it **"junk food"**. But even junk food is still edible. Our twentieth century lifestyle is far removed from the life of a first century orthodox Jew. Paul, the writer of the book of Romans, was a first century Hebrew, a Pharisee, and a rabbi schooled very extensively in the Scriptures. To Paul, when words like **"clean"**, **"pure"**, or **"legal"** were spoken in relationship to food, the supreme authority on such dietary matters was **always** the Word of God—the Holy Scriptures. **To the apostle Paul, food only refered to those items outlined by God in His word!** Since the Word of God calls shrimp, lobster, crab, pork, rabbit, and other creatures listed in Deuteronomy 14 and Leviticus 11 unclean or not edible, these would not be considered as food to Paul. To anyone who obeyed God's word, the **"SHALT**

101

NOT" list of animals, fish, birds, and creeping things was considered detestable, abominable, unhealthy, impure and unclean to touch, much less to eat. Since it is clear in Scripture that God calls certain creatures unclean, what did Paul mean when he said in Romans 14:14 that there is nothing unclean of itself? To rightly divide and understand Paul's comments, it would be helpful to look at I Corinthians chapters 8 and 10 since the same issue of foods offered to idols is addressed.

I CORINTHIANS CHAPTERS 8 AND 10

The eating of "unclean" things is forbidden in God's word. **Unclean things are not edible!** Therefore, when Paul uses the words, "the eating of things offered to idols," he is referring to "clean" foods. What about "clean foods" offered to idols? Should believers eat clean foods offered to idols? Paul addresses this problem when he wrote:

"Therefore, concerning the eating of things offered to idols, we know that an idol is nothing in the world and that there is no other God but one. For even if there are so called gods.......yet for us there is only one God, the Father, of whom are all things, and we for Him; and one Lord Jesus Christ, through whom are all things, and through whom we live."

(I Corinthians 8:4-6)

Paul is confirming in I Corinthians 8:4-6 that we should have no other gods before the God of Abraham, Isaac, and Jacob because He is supreme; the Creator of all things and the giver of life. All other gods are nothing in comparison with the one true and Almighty God. Paul continues:

"However, there is not in everyone that knowledge; for some with consciousness of the idol, until now eat it as things offered to an idol; and their conscience, being weak, is defiled."
(I Corinthians 8:7)

Paul realizes that there are brothers and sisters who don't understand the awesomeness of God and give power to these pagan gods, fearing the demons associated with the idols. These **"weaker"** brothers, as Paul refers to them, refuse these clean foods offered to the idols because of the fear of being **"defiled"** by them.

The knowledge of the authority and supremacy of God over demons was not yet fully comprehended by some in the early church. Paul is stating a phenomena true of some in the Church today. Some people fear satan's power more than the power and authority of Yeshua (Jesus) to overcome any power satan or his demons may "try" to exercise over them. Paul continues by ephasizing that eating foods offered to idols in the presence of a "weaker" brother might cause him to stumble or even fall away from the faith:

"And because of your knowledge shall the weak brother perish, for whom Christ died?"
(I Corinthians 8:11)

Paul concludes I Corinthians chapter 8 by stating that he is willing to stop eating clean meat, even if the Word of God permits it, in order that a brother may not stumble or fall because of his actions.

*"Therefore, if food makes my brother stumble,
I will never eat meat, lest I make
my brother stumble."*
(I Corinthians 8:13)

Paul is referring to clean meat in this passage since
unclean meat is never considered by a Jew like Paul to be
"food". Refusing to eat clean meat in order to keep a
brother from "stumbling" is not going against the Word of
God. However, eating unclean foods in order to keep a
brother from stumbling would be contrary to the Scriptures.

Paul continues the theme of foods (clean of course)
offered to idols in chapter 10 of I Corinthians:

*"What am I saying then? That an idol is any-
thing, or what is offered to idols anything?"*
(I Corinthians 10:19)

Paul again emphasizes that God is supreme and that
food offered to idols has no real authority over the name of
Jesus. If a believer eats these clean foods offered to idols,
they have not broken God's commands. This next statement by Paul has been misinterpreted for almost two
thousand years and has given license for many to unknowingly violate the Word of God:

*"All things are lawful for me, but all things are not
helpful; all things are lawful for me;
but all things do not edify."*
(I Corinthians 10:23)

Is Paul giving us permission to murder, commit adultery, lie, steal, and eat unclean things? God forbid! When

Paul says the word **"lawful",** he means those things allowed by God in His word. The Word of God prohibits idolatry, adultery, stealing, eating unclean things, as well as many other things. These actions are **"unlawful"** or forbidden. Paul is explaining that even though he is not forbidden to eat clean things offered to idols in God's word, he can still cause a brother to fall away by eating these things and this does not edify his brother. In **I Corinthians 6:12** Paul repeats these very words that **"all things are lawful for me, but all things are not helpful"** and continues in the next verse to empasize the important point that our bodies belong to God. He also wants us to remember, as Jesus explains in Matthew 15 and Mark 7 that both food and our bodies will pass away:

"Foods for the stomach and the stomach for foods, but God will destroy both it and them. Now the body is not for sexual immorality but for the Lord, and the Lord for the body"
(I Corinthians 6:13)

Paul emphasizes that our body is for the Lord and the Lord is for our body. The Lord desires for us to do what is lawful for our body, that is to be obedient to His word. His word covers every aspect of a holy life, including eating healthy foods. God's word is always for our well being, but we should also consider the well being of others:

"Let no one seek his own, but each other's well being."
(I Corinthians 10:24)

These next two passages of Scripture have been quoted, out of their context, to encourage people to eat whatever is placed before you. But Paul, keeper of God's word, is saying throughout these passages that the Word does not prohibit us from eating clean meats offered to idols, but we should eat them without making an issue out of whether this or that clean meat has been offered to an idol:

"Eat whatever is sold in the meat market, asking no questions....."
(I Corinthians 10:25)

We must remember that a Jew, like Paul, when entering a Gentile meat market would pass right by the shrimp, lobster, and pork. Paul is suggesting that when a believer finds himself in a heathen or Gentile meat market, such as in Rome or Corinth (where idols were worshipped), he should not inquire of the butcher or salesperson whether the clean meat was offered to idols. Just buy and enjoy. He gives the same advice to a believer invited to an unbeliever's home for dinner:

"If any of those who do not believe invites you to dinner, and you desire to go, eat whatever is set before you, asking no questions...."
(I Corinthians 10:27)

The phrase, **"eat whatever is set before you"**, would include **only** the edible or clean foods outlined in the Scriptures. Paul is telling us not to be concerned whether these **"edible"** foods were offered to strange gods.

BACK TO ROMANS 14

Now we can understand Romans 14 in its **proper context** - According to Paul, the foods that God has declared clean can not be made unclean when offered to idols. But, "to him who considers anything to be unclean, to him it is unclean." (Romans 14:14) One person believes he can eat all **(clean)** meats offered to idols and another, afraid of defilement by the idol, refuses to eat meat (being weak in the faith) and eats only vegetables. The Scriptures are silent about whether we should eat meats offered to idols; therefore, Paul urges us not to argue over "doubtful things."

"Receive one who is weak in the faith, but not to disputes over doubtful things. For one believes he may eat all things, but he who is weak eats only vegetables. Let not him who eats despise him who does not eat, and let him who does not eat judge him who eats; for God has received him."

(Romans 14:1-3)

Paul is convinced by Jesus Himself that whatever God has declared in His word to be clean to eat, is clean, and no idol can make it unclean. To believe that an idol can defile what God has declared to be clean would be giving more authority to the idol than to God. Yet, for those who believe that strange gods can defile what God has declared clean, Paul suggests they should not eat such things:

"I know and am convinced by the Lord Jesus that there is nothing unclean of itself; but to him who considers anything to be unclean, to him it is unclean."

(Romans 14:14)

Paul reaffirms what he said in I Corinthians 10 about abstaining from clean or pure meats offered to idols if it would cause a brother to be offended and to stumble:

"Do not destroy the work of God for the sake of food. All things indeed are pure, but it is evil for a man who eats with offense. It is good neither to eat meat nor drink wine nor do anything by which your brother stumbles or is offended or is made weak."
(Romans 14:20-21)

The Word of God concerning pure foods, or any other teaching of the Bible must be received and understood by faith. If anyone eats these clean or pure foods offered to idols and is not fully convinced in his heart that the idols can not harm him, then doubt has opened the door to satan:

"But he who doubts is condemned if he eats, because he does not eat from faith; for whatever is not of faith is sin."
(Romans 14:23)

If the eating of clean meats offered to idols was contrary to the Word of God, Paul would have rebuked those in error. But God's word is silent on this matter and so Paul admonishes us, "not to dispute over doubtful things" (Romans 14:1). Shall we in the Church dispute over doubtful points of doctrine upon which the Scriptures are either silent or vague? **Let us instead restore to the Church God's dietary principles upon which the Scriptures are neither vague nor silent!**

ENTERING THE KINGDOM OF GOD

As important as clean foods are in building and maintaining a strong and healthy temple for God's Holy Spirit to dwell in, following God's dietary principles does not give us access to the kingdom of God. **A person can only enter the kingdom of God by grace through faith in Jesus as Lord and Messiah and the receiving of God's Holy Spirit.** Paul emphasizes this important point:

"For the kingdom of God is not food and drink, but righteousness and peace and joy in the Holy Spirit."
(Romans 14:17)

Many false doctrines, especially at the time of Jesus, insisted that food could defile us spiritually and Jesus dealt with this wrong teaching in Matthew 15 and Mark 7. Food can not defile us spiritually, but it can most certainly harm us physically.

FOOD DOES NOT DEFILE US SPIRITUALLY
(MARK 7 AND MATTHEW 15)

"There is nothing that enters a man from outside which can defile him; but the things that come out of him, those are the things that defile him."
(Mark 7:15)

"Not what goes into the mouth defiles a man;
but what comes out of the mouth,
this defiles a man."
(Matthew 15:11)

Is Jesus saying in these two passages that food can not defile or harm our physical bodies when we have seen and read so much in the media about high fat diets full of cholesterol contributing to higher rates of heart disease and cancer? What we eat can most certainly defile our body, but food does not commend us to God (I Corinthians 8:8). Jesus was addressing the condition of our spiritual heart, not our physical heart.

INTENT OF THE HEART

In both Matthew 15:11 and Mark 7:15, Jesus was responding to the Pharisees who insisted that His disciples were eating with unwashed hands and therefore were defiling themselves spiritually.

"Why do your disciples transgress the tradition of
the elders? For they do not wash their hands
when they eat bread."
(Matthew 15:2)

According to Jewish ceremonial law, a person who ate before washing his hands defiled himself. Ceremonial washing was an oral **tradition of the elders,** not a **commandment of God** written in the Scriptures. This man-made commandment was not for hygiene purposes but it was done for the purpose of spiritual purity. The religious Jews of Jesus' time had the false belief that physical cleanliness brought spiritual cleanliness, but only the blood of Jesus can make a person spiritually clean. They were not able to see or willing to admit the wickedness that existed within their own hearts and the need for a Savior to deliver them from their inner life of sin. Following any outward religious practice such as reading the Bible, attending church, tithing, or eating clean foods does not make us spiritually clean before God. God is looking within us at the condition of our heart towards Him. **Jesus was not concerned with the cleanliness of a man's hands, but the cleanness of a man's heart.** He used the accusation of the Pharisees as an opportunity to teach the difference between outward religious observances and the inward spiritual condition of the heart. Jesus quoted the prophet Isaiah to the Pharisees concerning the condition of their hearts.

"These people draw near to Me with their mouth, and draw near to Me with their lips, but their heart is far from Me. And in vain they worship Me, teaching as doctrines the commandments of men."
(Matthew 15:8-9)

God, speaking through Isaiah, tells us in this passage that the outward actions of a person may look religious, but their **heart** may be far from God. When God looks at our heart, He sees our motives. The Pharisees wore religious garments, followed man-made religious rituals, and prayed long religious prayers not because they loved God, but because they wanted to be seen, heard, and revered by men.

> *"Every way of a man is right in his own eyes,*
> *But the Lord weighs the hearts."*
> *(Proverbs 21:2)*

God is not impressed with outward appearances; He looks at the heart. The Lord told the prophet Samuel:

> *"....For the Lord does not see as a man sees;*
> *for man looks at the outward appearance,*
> *but the Lord looks at the heart."*
> *(I Samuel 16:7)*

In Matthew 15 and Mark 7 Jesus is teaching that **spiritual defilement is a matter of what comes out of the heart, not what goes into the body.** His disciples did not understand this teaching, so Jesus gave them a physiology lesson in Matthew 15:17 and the following Scripture:

> *"Are you thus without understanding also? Do*
> *you not perceive that whatever enters a man*
> *from outside can not defile him, because it does*
> *not enter his heart but his stomach, and is*
> *eliminated, thus purifying all foods."*
> *(Mark 7:18-19)*

Some versions of the Bible set apart "thus purifying all foods" as Mark's comment on what Jesus was saying. Biblical scholars have interpreted Mark's comment to mean that Jesus declared all foods clean, when in fact, Mark was merely expressing his understanding of Jesus' comment on digestion and elimination. Digestion is the process by which the body breaks down food into useable nutrients - proteins, carbohydrates, fats, vitamins, and minerals. After digestion occurs, the unusable portions of food must be eliminated otherwise they would pollute the internal organs and blood. Thus elimination is the way the body cleanses or purifies itself.

Nowhere in these verses does Jesus declare all foods to be clean. Clean and unclean foods are not even an issue in these Scriptures. We must remember that the Jews ate only what had been set apart or sanctified by God as food. The discussion is about whether eating food with unwashed hands can defile a man spiritually. Jesus was telling his disciples that eating food with dirty hands doesn't defile a man. A man defiles himself by the evil that comes out of his heart.

"But those things which proceed out of the mouth come from the heart, and they defile a man. For out of the heart proceed evil thoughts, murders, adulteries, fornications, thefts, false witness, blasphemies. These are the things which defile a man, but to eat with unwashed hands does not defile a man."
(Matthew 15:18-20)

We take care of our temple by following the nutritional principles of the Bible because we love God and want to be good stewards of the body He has given to us; not to become more spiritual. If we do not obey these principles, it won't keep us from going to Heaven, in fact, it may get us there sooner!

113

SHOULD GENTILES KEEP THE DIETARY COMMANDS?
(ACTS 15)

"For it seemed good to the Holy Spirit, and to us, to lay no greater burden than these necessary things: that you abstain from things offered to idols, from blood, from things strangled, and from fornication. If you keep yourselves from these, you will do well."
(Acts 15:28-29)

SIMPLICITY OF THE GOSPEL

The apostles in Acts 15 did not want to give the new Gentile believers overwhelming rules to follow because they wanted to emphasize the simplicity of the salvation message; that is, **the free gift of God is eternal life in Jesus Christ.** The purpose for which Acts 15 was written is stated in the first verse:

"And certain men came down from Judea and taught the brothern, 'Unless you are circumcised according to the custom of Moses, you can not be saved.' "
(Acts 15:1)

The issue is simply—**Do you have to keep the law to be saved**? Obviously, the answer is no! Salvation is

114

not received by works of the law. **Yeshua alone brings salvation**. For we are saved by grace through faith in the Lord Jesus Christ. It is not of works least any man should boast. But some of the believing Pharisees said:

"....It is necessary to circumcise them, and to command them to keep the law of Moses.

So the apostles and elders came together

to consider the matter."

(Acts 15:5-6)

Peter addresses the assembly about this issue by reminding them of what happened to Cornelius, his family, and his Gentile friends (Acts 10):

"....that by my mouth the Gentiles should hear the word of the gospel and believe. So God, who knows the heart, acknowledged them by giving them the Holy Spirit just as He did to us and made no distinction between us and them, purifying their hearts by faith. Now therefore, why do you test God by putting a yoke on the neck of the disciples which neither our fathers nor we were able to bear? But we believe through the grace of the Lord Jesus we shall be saved in the same manner as they."

(Acts 15:7-11)

The leader of the congregation in Jerusalem agreed with Peter's comments (Acts 15:13-19) and the whole assembly decided to write a letter to the new Gentile converts who were troubled in their souls by the message that they had to keep the law to be saved. The Gentiles to whom they were writing were coming out of pagan temple worship and knew nothing of the Holy Scriptures. The elders at Jerusalem did not want to trouble the Gentiles who were turning to God but they wrote to them to abstain from idol worship, from temple prostitution or sexual immorality, from things strangled, and from drinking blood sacrifices. As a beginning, if they kept themselves from these, they would be doing well in their new life in Christ.

The first century Jewish apostles understood that although the path to salvation is very narrow, it would be very discouraging in the beginning for new converts to know just how much their lives would have to change as they followed Jesus. The words **"no greater burden"** in these verses are vital to understanding the context of Acts 15. In the city of Corinth, Paul was dealing with a society of pagan worship and immorality. His first and foremost concern was always with a person's salvation, then putting a stop to their pagan practices and teaching them God's commandments.

Were these four **"necessary things"** in Acts 15:28-29 all that the Gentiles would ever have to do? Of course not! The apostles knew that these first century Gentile converts would eventually be taught: to love their neighbor as themselves, to honor their father and mother, not to steal, not to bear false witness, to take care of their temple (by keeping the dietary laws), as well as the other commandments of the one true God. The apostles in Acts 15 knew that these "babies in Christ" would study God's word, the Law and the Prophets, and begin to drink the pure milk of the Word, as they attended the synagogues:

*"For Moses has had throughout many generations
those who preach him in every city,
being read in the synagogues."
(Acts 15:21)*

The Lord gave us certain foods to heal, restore, and maintain our temples so we can fullfill His will and purpose for our lives. He made a distinction in foods between the clean and the unclean, but when it comes to salvation He makes no distinctions. **Whosoever** will come to the waters of repentence and accept Jesus as Lord and Savior can receive the free gift of eternal life. **God sent His Son, Yeshua, to reconcile us to Himself.** It doesn't matter what we have done, what we have accomplished, or what we have failed to accomplish; it is Jesus who justifies each of us before the Father by His blood which was shed on the cross and sprinkled over our lives. Eternal life is found in the blood, the blood of Jesus.

JUDGE NOT
IN FOOD OR DRINK
(COLOSSIANS 2:16)

*"So let no one judge you in food or drink,
or regarding a festival or a new moon or sabbaths,
which are a shadow of things to come,
but the substance is of Christ."
(Colossians 2:16-17)*

In this Scripture, Paul is not giving us permission to eat contrary to the Word of God, he is warning the Colossians not to let anyone judge them concerning their salvation on the basis of what they eat or drink. Paul is addressing a problem that arose in the predominantly Gentile church at Colosse which combined the elements of Greek philosophy (Colossians 2:4,8-10), Jewish legalism (Colossians 2:11-17), and Oriental mysticism (Colossians 2: 18-23) which taught that their salvation and right standing with God was dependent upon following certain religious practices. This type of religious system was threatening the Colossian church. Paul was dealing with the same issues as in Matthew 15, Mark 7, and Acts 15 - **religious traditions** and **salvation through works.** Attempting to fit Jesus into any religious system which requires works for salvation undermines His redemptive work.

"Beware lest anyone cheat you through philosophy and empty deceit, according to the traditions of men, according to the basic principles of the world, and not according to Christ."

(Colossians 2:8)

Until God sent His Son, Yeshua, believers were trying to follow God's commandments in order to be righteous and attain good standing with Him. We could not keep all of God's regulations set forth in His word because of the weakness of our flesh and we remained dead spiritually and separated from His promises. The righteous requirements of God's word were kept fully by Yeshua while He lived in a physical body and His sacrifice on the cross removed the judgement against us all:

*"having wiped out the handwriting of requirements
that was against us, which was contrary to us.
And he has taken it out of the way,
having nailed it to the cross."*
(Colossians 2:14)

The principles of the world are directly opposed to the principles of Christ. The principles of Christ always line up with the Word of God. The **"basic principles of the world"** refer to religious practices that force a person back into works in order to earn salvation and right standing with God. Believers at Colosse were being condemned by religious people for not keeping the "law of Moses". They were being told that they needed to do certain religious practices in order to be saved and were being judged as unsaved if they did not. (see Colossians 2:16-17 above). Paul warned the Colossians not to be deceived by these false teachers and false teachings:

*"Let no man defraud you of your reward, taking
delight in false humility and worship of angels,
intruding into those things which he has not seen,
vainly puffed up by his fleshly mind,
and not holding fast to the Head...."*
(Colossians 2:18-19)

Paul reminds the Colossians that they should not get sidetracked with man-made religious works in order to become accepted by God:

119

"Therefore, if you died with Christ from the basic principles of the world, why, as though living in the world, do you subject yourselves to regulations - 'Do not touch, do not taste, do not handle, which all concern things which perish with the using - according to the commandments and doctrines of men?"
(Colossians 2:20-22)

The dietary commands of the Bible are neither doctrines of men nor basic principles of the world; they are the instructions of God. The **"commandments and doctrines of men"** are self-imposed religious practices that originate in the world not the Spirit. Paul tells us that such rituals are earthly and feed our flesh rather than our spirits.

"These things indeed have an appearance of wisdom in self-imposed religion, false humility, and neglect of the body, but are of no value against the indulgence of the flesh."
(Colossians 2:23)

We are in right standing with the Lord, not because of something we have done, such as following His regulations, but because of what Jesus did for us. We stand in His righteousness. Do we still keep His word? Of course we do! But our motive has changed from trying to be righteous and acceptable to God, to gratefully following His instructions because we love Him. We are to follow the Word of God and not the doctrines of men.

To eat according to Biblical nutrition is not **"neglect of the body"** or an a **"indulgence of the flesh".** On the contrary, it is good stewardship of the body that God has given us and enables us to continue seeking the things which are above:

"If you were raised with Christ, seek those things which are above, where Christ is, sitting at the right hand of God......Therefore put to death your members which are on the earth: fornication, uncleanness, passion, evil desire, and covetousness, which is idolatry."
(Colossians 3:1,5)

Following God's nutritional principles because we love Him is of value "against the indulgence of the flesh". When we purpose in our hearts, as Daniel did, not to eat the deceptive foods of the world, but rather the wholesome foods of God, we put to death one of the desires of our flesh.

"And those who are Christ's have crucified the flesh with its passions and desires."
(Galatians 5:24)

121

CHAPTER SIX

FASTING FOR HEALTH
SPIRITUAL AND PHYSICAL RENEWAL

*"Is this not the fast that I have chosen: To loose
the bonds of wickedness, to undue the heavy
burdens, to let the oppressed go free,
And that you break every yoke?"
(Isaiah 58:6)*

Fasting is more than abstaining from all solid food or certain foods for a period of time, it is a way to "humble ourselves" (Psalm 35:13) before the Lord and seek His face. In chapter 58 of the book of Isaiah, the Lord rebukes Israel for fasting with selfish motives instead of interceding for the needs of others. God directs us to fast on behalf of the oppressed, those laden with heavy burdens, and for those who are in slavery in their spirit, soul, or body. He encourages us to share the food we would have eaten with the hungry and minister to the poor. **Fasting is a powerful act on our part to put aside "our flesh" and its desires in order to reach out to others.** God promises us that if we fast with our attention upon the needs of others, that He will meet our needs as well:

"If you extend your soul to the hungry and satisfy the afflicted soul, then your light shall dawn in the darkness, and your darkness shall be as the noonday. The Lord will guide you continually, and satisfy you in draught, and strengthen your bones; You shall be like a watered garden, and like a spring of water, whose waters do not fail."
(Isaiah 58:11)

As we turn away from our needs with fasting and prayer for the concerns of others, the Lord promises to strengthen, heal, and encourage us as well. As we fast according to God's purposes He says that we will be called the "repairer of the breach and the restorer of streets to dwell in" (Isaiah 58:12). God gives us the opportunity through prayer and fasting to take part in the ministry of our Lord Jesus who was the true "Repairer of the breach". Even now, Jesus reaches out to us who are poor and needy showing us the compassion and mercy of God. Fasting is an opportunity to say "no" to that part of us that says, "I", "Me", "Mine", and "My way!," and say "yes" to God's way.

Throughout history, prayer and fasting have played a significant part in the lives of the men and women God has used to influence the destiny of the Church. Fasting is not a discipline conceived in the mind of a man, but by God Himself:

"Now, therefore, says the Lord, Turn to Me
with all your heart, with fasting,
with weeping, and with mourning."
(Joel 2:12)

Abraham fasted, Moses fasted, Daniel fasted, the first
century church fasted, and even the Son of God fasted.
Jesus began His ministry with a forty day fast in which
He overcame temptation in the same three areas that
caused man to fall. **The first Adam fell by eating; the
last Adam (Jesus) overcame by fasting!**

1. Satan said, "If You are the Son of God, command
that these stones become bread." Jesus said to him,
**"Man shall not live by bread alone, but by every
word that proceeds from the mouth of God"
(Matthew 4:4, Deuteronomy 8:3).** Jesus was a man
under authority; the authority of God His Father. In
the gospel of John, Jesus says: **"For I have not spoken on My own authority; but the Father who
sent Me gave Me a command, what I should say
and what I should speak. And I know that His
command is everlasting life. Therefore, whatever I speak, just as the Father has told Me, so I
speak."** (John 12: 49-50) Jesus was hungry, but
God had not commanded Him to change the stones
into bread. He honored only the commands of His
Father which bring life, not those of satan which bring
death. Man "saw that the tree was good for food"
(Genesis 3:6) and ate of it against God's command thus
bringing death into the world.

2. Satan said, "If You are the Son of God, throw yourself down." He quoted Psalm 91:11-12 and told Jesus
that He would not be harmed because God's angels
would protect Him. Jesus responded, **"You shall not**

tempt the Lord your God" (Matthew 4:7, Deuteronomy 6:16). Jesus only did those things He saw His Father do. He knew that His Father's commands brought life and that Satan's temptations brought death. The serpent told man he would not die if he ate of the tree of the knowledge of good and evil, but God said he would. Man, being tempted by satan, disobeyed God thus resulting in death, but Jesus obeyed His Father and brought life. **"For since by a man came death, by a man also came the resurrection of the dead." (I Corinthians 15:21)**

3. Satan showed Jesus all the kingdoms of the world and their glory and said, "All these things I will give You if You will fall down and worship me." Jesus responded, **"You shall worship the Lord your God, and Him alone shall you serve" (Matthew 4:10, Deuteronomy 6:13).** Satan promised Jesus all the power, riches, and authority that this world had to offer, but Jesus knew that all authority had <u>already</u> been given to Him in heaven <u>and on earth</u> (Matthew 28:18). The word worship means to show great honor and respect. Jesus knew that all honor, respect, and glory belonged to His Father. Satan led man to believe that if he ate of the tree he would be like God possessing God's wisdom. There is no wisdom, power, or authority apart from God. By eating of the tree, man bowed down and honored satan's word above God's word.

Just as Jesus triumphed through His perfect obedience where Adam and Eve fell through their disobedience, He also triumphed where the children of Israel were disobedient. Moses was commanded by God to place three things into the Ark of the Covenant as a **"testimony against"** the children of Israel (Hebrews 9:4, Deuteronomy 31:26-

27, Numbers 17:10, Numbers 11:1-4):

1. **manna** - The children of Israel complained about God's provision and desired other food. But Jesus said to satan, "...man shall not live by bread alone; but man lives by every word that proceeds from the mouth of the Lord." (Deuteronomy 8:3)

2. **Aaron's rod** - Aaron's rod was a symbol of the authority of God that the children of Israel tested and rebelled against. Jesus never tested the authority of His Father and said to satan, "You shall not tempt the Lord your God..." (Deuteronomy 6:16).

3. **tablets of the covenant** - The children of Israel worshipped the golden calf and broke the first two commandments. Jesus said to satan, "You shall fear (worship) the Lord your God and serve Him..." (Deuteronomy 6:13).

When Jesus was tempted by satan, He countered the **"testimony against"** Israel by His perfect obedience to the Word of God.

JESUS INSTRUCTS US TO FAST

There is no question about whether we should fast because our Lord said, **"when you fast."**

"Moreover, when you fast, do not be like the hypocrites, with a sad countenance."
(Matthew 6:16)

Jesus was telling us that there would come a time when we would fast. Later in Matthew 9:15, Jesus, our bridegroom, tells us <u>when</u> we will fast:

"..But the days will come when the bridegroom will be taken away from them, and then they will fast."
(Matthew 9:15)

From the time that Jesus was taken into heaven two thousand years ago, until the time He returns again in glory, believers everywhere have been called to fast.

PRAYER AND FASTING

Prayer and fasting is an act of worship that ministers to the Lord **(Acts 13:2)**. Just as a hunger strike gets man's attention, prayer and fasting draws God's attention. Prayer and fasting says you have a hunger for God that is greater than your physical desire to eat.

The Bible gives us many spiritual reasons to fast. In Ezra 8:21 we are given three excellent purposes for fasting: 1. to seek direction for our life, 2. to seek direction for family members, and 3. to seek direction for finances, business, or investments.

"Then I proclaimed a fast...that we might humble ourselves before our God, to seek from Him the right way for us and our little ones and all our possessions."

The book of Esther establishes another reason for prayer and fasting - **to intercede for a people or a nation**. Esther and the Jewish people fasted for God to intervene in the affairs of their nation in order to stop the plot to annihilate the Jewish people.

"Go, gather all the Jews who are present in Shushan, and fast for me; neither eat nor drink for three days, night or day. My maids and I will fast likewise."
(Esther 4:16)

King David, "a man after God's own heart", fasted for his dying child.

"So he said, 'While the child was still alive, I
fasted and wept; for I said, Who can tell
whether the Lord will be gracious to me,
that the child may live"
(II Samuel 12:22)

In the book of Jonah, a whole city fasted as an act of repentance:

"So the people of Nineveh believed God,
proclaimed a fast, and put on sackcloth,
from the greatest to the least of them."
(Jonah 3:5)

The prophet Daniel fasted and repented for his nation:

"Then I set my face toward the Lord God
to make request by prayer and supplications,
with fasting, sackcloth, and ashes."
(Daniel 9:3)

A few more Biblical reasons to fast include:
1. Ministering to the Lord (Acts 13:2)
2. For others less fortunate (Isaiah 58:6)
3. Equipping people for ministry (Matthew 4:1)

Fasting is not an option, it's a necessity! Most important of all, fasting helps us to grow closer to God and to hear His voice, but fasting is also helpful to our physical body as well. Cleansing the body of toxins in order to bring healing and rejuvenation are some of the **physical benefits** of fasting.

CLEANSING THE TEMPLE

Your body is a temple of the Lord where His Holy Spirit dwells (I Corinthians 6:19). The Lord has a very exact plan for the proper care of your temple. His plan includes eating a high complex carbohydrate, high fiber, low protein, low sodium, and low fat diet (Genesis 1:29, Leviticus 3:16-17, Leviticus 11, and Deuteronomy 14). Unfortunately, most of us have saturated our bodies with greasy and sugary foods that are full of pesticides, chemicals, parasites, artificial flavors, and artificial colors. We have also introduced poisonous medicines, drugs, and vaccines into our bodies over the course of a lifetime. So what can we do to rid our bodies of all these potentially harmful toxins? We can fast! Fasting is an excellent way to cleanse your system, if done properly. Of all nature's techniques for healing your body, fasting is one of the most effective. Eliminating solid food and drinking fluids instead, permits the body to muster all its resoures for "cleaning the house" instead of digesting food. The therapeutic effect of fasting has been well documented by many years of clinical experience both in Europe and in the United States. Fasting is an opportunity for a "new beginning" to recuperate, renew, and regroup lost energy and health.

Just as the priests of old went into a physical building that had been neglected for many years and cleaned out all of the garbage that had been put there, so the priests of today, the body of Messiah, can cleanse their "temples" physically:

"Then the priests went into the inner part of the house of the Lord to cleanse it, and brought out all the debris that they found in the temple of the

Lord to the court of the house of the Lord. And the Levites took it out and carried it to the Brook Kidron."
(II Chronicles 29:16)

AUTOINTOXICATION

Autointoxication is self-poisoning of all or part of the body by the internal accumulation of toxic matter. Many people are sick because of **autointoxication**. It is a form of slow suicide! When done through ignorance, it is unintentional suicide and when done because of stubbornness, it is intentional suicide!

Detoxification is the removing of toxic materials collected over the years from bad diet, poor health habits, and the environment. Symptoms of toxic overload include headaches, joint pain, digestive problems, low energy, allergic reactions, anxiety, depression, and mental confusion. We can choose to detoxify or cleanse these poisons by different types of fasting.

The prophet Jeremiah was set over the nations by the Lord. Before Jeremiah could "build and plant", he had to "root out....destroy....and throw down."

"To root out and pull down, To destroy and to throw down, To build and to plant."
(Jeremiah 1:10)

When waxing a floor, you must first strip the old wax off before applying the new wax. Similiarly, before anyone can expect to build or regain health, it is usually necessary to tear down and eliminate the old debris from the body first. **Fasting is a "tearing down" process**

where the body uses all of its energy to eliminate the "the debris" or accumulated toxins from the internal organs, arteries, and blood. After this detoxification or cleansing takes place, then you can rebuild by eating **The Genesis Diet**.

DANGERS OF FASTING

When properly done, fasting will result in physical, mental, and spiritual invigoration! Fasting done incorrectly and for the wrong reasons can be dangerous and unhealthy. Fasting in order to drop fifteen to forty pounds in a month or six weeks damages the endocrine glands (especially the thyroid), the sexual hormones, and your metabolism. **Starving is not fasting!** Such a quick, unhealthy, weight loss leaves a person's body depleted and exhausted. A slow, progressive weight loss of two pounds per week is the healthiest and safest way to experience permanent weight loss (see **Breaking the Fat Barrier**). Fasting to achieve quick weight loss is as unhealthy as using cigarettes for weight loss.

Also, fasting without fluids, as Moses did, is very dangerous, unless you are in God's presence continually, as Moses was. You can exist without solid food for forty or more days, but only seven days without fluids! To fast without food or water for forty days is not natural, it's supernatural!

If you have a diagnosed illness and/or are taking drugs, fasting should only be done under the direct supervision of a health practitioner. Some people who have trouble fasting because they have undiagnosed low blood sugar become extremely hungry, dizzy, and nauseous and should drink fruit and vegetable juices to help keep the blood sugar stable during short fasts.

HOW TO BEGIN AND END

There are specific ways to prepare for and break a fast. Fasts of one to three days usually do not require any special preparation. However, fasts of three days or more should be preceeded by two or more days of eating raw fruits and vegetables. Fasts of three days or more should never be broken by eating a normal meal because these heavy foods put a severe strain and shock on the digestive organs which have been resting throughout the fast. It is not uncommon to see people come off a fast and binge on their favorite junk foods for weeks. Breaking fasts with a pound of fruit such as grapes is a gentle way to reintroduce solid food into the digestive system and also helps stimulate a natural bowel movement. Eat raw fruits and vegetables for one to three days after the fast before adding heavier foods such as animal proteins back into the diet.

WHAT TO DRINK

To help the kidneys eliminate the toxins from the body during a fast, drink approximately a gallon of liquid each day. Distilled water may be included as part of the fluids. Raw fruit juices such as orange and grapefruit (not recommended for arthritis or allergy sufferers), grape, pineapple, and apple are excellent providers of needed natural sugar to stablize the blood sugar and keep the energy level up. Raw vegetable juices such as carrot, celery, beet, or green vegetable combinations are excellent as well. Fresh fruit and vegetable juices can be made in a juice extractor. They provide excellent sources of amino acids (simple proteins), vitamins, minerals, trace minerals, beta carotene, chlorophyll, and phytochemicals in an easily digestable form. If a juice extractor is unavailable purchase fruit and vegtable juices without any added sugars.

Another important beverage used in European fasting clinics is **vegetable broth.** This potassium-rich drink is prepared as follows:

> 2 large potatoes, unpeeled, chopped or sliced to approximately one-half inch pieces
>
> 1 cup carrots, shedded or sliced
>
> 1 cup red beets, shredded or sliced
>
> 1 cup celery, leaves and all, chopped to one-half inch pieces
>
> 1 cup chopped onion
>
> 1 cup other vegetables: beet tops, turnips and tops, parsley, cabbage, or a little of everything

Use a stainless steel, enameled, or earthenware pot and fill it with one and one-half quarts of distilled water. Clean vegetables well, but do not peel. Cut all the vegetables directly into the water to prevent oxidation. Cover and cook slowly for at least a half an hour. Let stand for a half an hour then strain and remove all vegtables from the broth. Cool and serve. If not used immediately, keep refrigerated and warm it again before serving.

ELIMINATION DURING A FAST

There are four avenues of elimination for removing accumulated poisons and toxins in the body: the bowels, the kidneys, the lungs, and the skin. During a fast of three days or more take an herbal laxative before bedtime or an enema to eliminate solid waste products. The fruit juices, vegetable juices, broth and water will remove many toxins via the kidneys. If strength permits, walk a half an hour a day to cleanse the lungs as well as do some deep breathing, inhaling through the nose and exhaling through the mouth.

Since one-third of the waste products eliminated during a fast are removed via the skin, adequate bathing is essential. Use a body brush or luffa sponge prior to bathing to invigorate the skin and loosen dead cells.

Improper or insufficient removal of wastes during a fast can harm rather than help a body. Attention must be paid to these four avenues of elimination or these organs can accumulate further toxins.

SUGGESTED FASTING SCHEDULE

1. Upon rising drink 8 ounces of distilled water with half a lemon squeezed into it.

2. Body brush skin before a warm and cool alternating shower.

3. Breakfast: Hot vegetable broth drink

4. Walk 30 minutes

5. Between meals: Drink plenty of fruit and vegetable juices

6. Lunch: Hot vegetable broth drink

7. Between meals: Drink more fruit and vegetable juices

8. Dinner: Hot vegetable broth drink

9. Retire early after reading the Bible

10. Take an herbal laxative with 8 ounces of water or an enema before bed.

It is best to start with a one to three day fast before attempting longer fasts. Fasting to improve your health is an honorable reason to fast, but an even better reason is to say "yes" to God and His plan for your life.

CHAPTER SEVEN

GOD'S PHARMACY
(HERBS FOR HEALING)

"For the earth which drinks in the rain that often comes upon it, and bears herbs useful for those by whom it is cultivated, receives blessing from God;"
(Hebrews 6:7)

God has placed healing properties in the plants He created. Hippocrates was right when he proclaimed, "Let medicine be your food and let food be your medicine." God, who provided healthy foods for the prevention of illness, has also provided medicinal herbs with special healing properties. There are literally thousands of medicinal herbs all over the world that man has come to appreciate. Truly, herbs are Biblical medicine in its most natural form. These natural herbs from God's pharmacy are used for such purposes as: purifying the blood, regulating the menstrual cycle, moving the bowels, cleansing the liver, removing headaches, fighting infections, and even burying the dead. It has been said that God in His grace has provided at least one herb for every illness or biological imbalance that man, in his fallen state, suffers from.

"He causes the grass to grow for the cattle, And the herbs (vegetation) for the service of man."
(Psalm 104:14)

Everyone can improve his or her health by the timely use of one or more of these medicinal herbs. This chapter will familiarize you with a few of the more common and available healing herbs. Whether these herbs are mentioned directly in the Scriptures like aloe, garlic, and hyssop, or simply come under the general heading of **"herbs for the service of man"**, they are all an important part of God's Pharmacy.

The great prophets of the Bible, who lived close to the land, knew the healing properties of plants. For instance, in II Kings the prophet Isaiah used figs to heal King Hezekiah's boils:

"Then Isaiah said, 'Take a lump of figs.'
So they took and laid it on the boil,
and he recovered."
(II Kings 20:7)

King Hezekiah wept and prayed before the Lord, asking Him to heal his terminal illness. The Lord sent the prophet Isaiah and told him to use the fruit of a plant to heal Hezekiah. **The God of all creation uses natural healing as well as supernatural healing!** God gave man the figs and the wisdom to use them for the **"service of man"**.

COMMON HERBS FOR HEALTH

There are many fine medicinal herb books that list hundreds of varieties of herbs for health and healing; therefore, the following is only a portion of God's bountiful supply of healing plants available to you. The list of herbs and their medicinal properties is based on the historic use of the plants through the ages. In an age when disease is rampant and medical costs are sky-rocketing, it is comforting to know the Lord has provided plants and herbs that contain natural chemicals in their fruits, leaves, bark, seeds, and roots which can assist our bodies in the healing process.

Even after "a new heaven and a new earth" and the New Jerusalem descends out of heaven in Revelation 21, God still plans to use the healing properties of plants to heal the nations.

".....And the leaves of the tree were for
the healing of the nations."
(Revelation 22:2)

CAUTION IN USE OF HERBS

Very few cases of death caused by medicinal herbal preparations have ever been documented compared to the thousands of recorded deaths annually from prescription drugs; however, side effects with herbs are possible. Just because herbs are natural rather than synthetic does not mean that they are totally harmless. For instance, herbs that contain caffeine could be harmful to some people. Caffeine containing herbs include kola nut, mate, and guarana. Warnings by doctors against the use of caffeine during pregnancy, lactation, or by individuals with high blood pressure, gastric ulcers, heart disease, or stimulant sensitivities should also include the above herbs as well as coffee and black tea. Many obese people are also cautioned against the use of caffeine because excess weight brings with it high blood pressure, circulatory problems, diabetic tendencies, and heart stress. Stimulating the heart of a person already overburdened by fifty or a hundred pounds of excess weight is unwise and even dangerous. Ma huang or ephedra is the oldest cultivated medicinal plant and the compounds in it increase heart activity more than caffeine. A powerful stimulate herb, Ma huang contains "ephedrine", a chemical used in respiratory drugs like Primatene and Sutafed. Ma huang is not recommended for people with diabetes, thyroid problems or prostate disease as well as all conditions where caffeine is prohibited. If you are overweight or have heart problems, high blood pressure, diabetes, prostate problems, or any serious condition stay away from these herbal stimulants, especially when they are combined into one tablet or capsule.

When taking any medicinal herb, always follow dosage directions on the container or bottle unless under the supervision of a health practitioner. Generally, herbs should be taken for specific purposes, in certain dosages, and for specific lengths of time. However, there is a class of herbs, called **tonic herbs,** that can be taken continually with good effects throughout a person's life. These tonic herbs may help specific health problems, but they can also be used to tone the whole body. Such herbs are alfalfa, bee pollen, cayenne, dandelion, garlic, ginger, ginseng, licorice, parsley, sea vegetables like dulse, kelp, and other algae, and royal jelly. Other herbs are classified as **spices** to be used in cooking and are listed in Chapter Two. **Herbs are natural medicines from God's Pharmacy and must be taken with wisdom.**

"Their fruit will be for food,
and their leaves for medicine"
(Ezekiel 47:12)

COMMON HERBS
AND THEIR HISTORIC USES

ALFALFA - arthritis, provides chlorophyll, alkalizes body, detoxifies body, morning sickness

BARBERRY BARK - jaudice, improves appetite, laxative affect

BAYBERRY - congestion in nose and sinuses, strengthens female organs

BEE POLLEN - energy food, allergies, male hormones

BLACK COHOSH - female estrogen, menstrual cramps, childbirth pain relief

BLACK WALNUT - cleanses parasites, expels tapeworms

BLESSED THISTLE - strengthens heart and lungs, circulates blood

BUCKTHORN - rheumatism, gout

BURDOCK - blood purifier, diuretic

CAPSICUM - circulation, stops internal bleeding

CASCARA SAGRADA - chronic constipation, helps secretion of bile

CHAMOMILE - nerves, toothaches, muscle pain

CHAPARRAL - cleanser, blood purifier, acne

COMFREY ROOT - blood cleanser, stomach, bowel, and fractures

CORNSILK - kidney and bladder, painful urination

DANDELION - liver cleanser, diuretic, anemia (iron)

FENNEL - colic in babies, aids digestion

FENUGREEK - fevers, lubrication of intestines

GINGER - indigestion, circulation

GINSENG - male hormone, longevity, stimulant

HAWTHORNE - dilate blood vessels, strengthen heart muscle wall

HOPS - insomnia, shock, restlessness

HORSETAIL (SPRINGTIME) - growth of hair and fingernails, absorption of calcium

KELP - thyroid, nails, loss of hair, removing radiation

LICORICE ROOT - hypoglycemia (low blood sugar), adrenals, hormonal support

LOBELIA - asthma, epilepsy, muscle action

MULLEIN - breathing problems, hay fever, glandular swelling

PAPAYA - enzyme for digestion, gas or sour stomach

PARSLEY - source of potassium and vitamin B, diuretic

PSYLLIUM - colon cleanser, bulking agent

RED CLOVER - blood purifier, lymphatic system

RED RASPBERRY - dysentery, strengthen uterine walls

ROSEHIPS - source of natural vitamin C, infection fighter

√**ROSEMARY** - prevent baldness, miscarriages, obesity

SAGE - night sweats, expel worms in children

SARSAPARILLA - male hormone, rheumatism, psoriasis, gout

SAW PALMETTO - alcoholism, prostate, asthma

SLIPPERY ELM - mucus membranes, bowels, kidneys

VALERIAN ROOT - nervous disorders, headaches, promotes sleep, muscle twitching

WHITE WILLOW BARK - varicose veins, headaches, fever, loose teeth

YARROW - diarrhea, mucus membranes

YELLOW DOCK - blood purifier, cleanser, acne, high in iron

YUCCA - arthritis

Below are few favorites to keep in your medicine chest, just for good measure.

ALOE

Aloe vera is mentioned five times in the Bible (Numbers 24:6, Psalm 45:8, Proverbs 7:17, Song of Solomon 4:14, John 19:39). Aloe vera gel is approved by the FDA for the treatment of burns and minor skin problems. There is nothing more soothing and healing for a sunburn than aloe vera gel. It can be applied to muscles and joints for the relief of pain and soreness. Aloe has also been used internally for a variety of applications. It has been effective as a natural cleanser or tonic for the whole body. Cape aloe is used as a natural laxative for sluggish bowels. Aloe vera has been used for the healing of ulcers and stomach problems in general.

ECHINACEA ROOT

This herbal remedy grows wild on the Great Plains. Health experts are singing the praises of echinacea as a healing agent and booster of the immune system. Three decades of European research have proved that echinacea has significant anti-viral, anti-bacterial, anti-fungal, and anti-inflammatory properties.

This special plant from God's pharmacy can help lessen the severity and shorten the time of colds and sore throats and various respiratory ailments. It may be given to children since studies have proven its effectiveness and safety. It is well suited for those conditions that come and go like colds, sore throats, flu symptoms, inflammation, and respiratory congestion, rather than deeply rooted problems. Purchase the freeze-dried variety in capsules from a health foods store. Take 2 capsules every 3 hours for a few days. Although tinctures of echinacea (liquid form of herb) may be easier to administer to young children, be sure to buy only the alcohol-free tinctures. The alcohol in some echinacea tinctures may destroy the polysaccharides that stimulate the immune system.

GARLIC

Garlic is mentioned in the Bible (Numbers 11:5) as a staple of Egypt and long accepted for its antibiotic power (known as Russian penicillin during World War II). It is also known to lower total cholesterol and improve the ratio of "good" cholesterol (HDL's) to "bad" cholesterol (LDL's). Garlic reduces the body's production of fats, prevents blood clotting by thinning the blood, and improves sluggish circulation. It has also been used as a dewormer for both animals and humans. Garlic's active ingredient **allicin** is the "smelly" characteristic of the pungent herb. Eating one to two fresh, crushed garlic cloves a day is a good way to use the herb medicinally. If smell is offensive, buy deodorized garlic supplements with significant amounts of allicin still in tact.

GOLDEN SEAL ROOT

One plant used by our ancestors as a healing remedy was golden seal root. Today, the demand is so great for this herb that it is a commonly cultivated perennial. It is one of those plants that is added to many herbal formulations because it seems to help a wide range of problems. Its reported properties include use as a diuretic, laxative, tonic, antiseptic, and astringent. It is used in stomach, intestinal, and liver disorders. As a tea, made from the powdered root, it can brushed on sore gums and teeth. Golden seal root has been helpful for mouth problems like pyorrhea and mouth ulcers or canker sores.

Golden seal root has the ability to dry up conditions where excess mucus is being manufactured such as with allergies, colds, and flus. Chronic catarrh (inflammation with discharge) is helped by this herb. The root contains **berberine**, an antibiotic useful against bacteria and fungi. Golden seal root should be taken in the same way and with the same caution as synthetic antibiotics because prolonged usage or high dosage of this herb may cause nausea, vomiting, a weakening of the bacterial flora of the colon, and a decreased white blood cell count. The best way to take golden seal root is in freeze-dried capsules - 2 capsules every 4 to 6 hours for five to seven days.

MINERALS AND TRACE MINERALS

"And God formed man from the dust of the ground and breathed into his nostrils the breath of life; and man became a living being."
(Genesis 2:7)

Man's body is made of many elements: oxygen, carbon, hydrogen, nitrogen, calcium, potassium, phosphorous, sulphur, chlorine, magnesium, iron, iodine, zinc and many other trace minerals. Since our bodies come from the soil, it is logical to assume that we need to take into our bodies the elements of the soil. Man sees himself as a very independent creature, yet his body is dependent upon the elements of the soil that God made him from.

At one time in America's history we had several feet of lush top soil; but today only a few inches remain. Where as the minerals and trace minerals in the soil were plentiful even a hundred years ago, today they are depleted. **Instead of replenishing the elements of the soil, we spread mineral deficient fertilizers on the little top soil remaining.** Many minerals and trace minerals which man at one time received through his food supply are simply not available in commercial fruits, vegetables, and grains. We need these elements from the soil, which are taken in by plants, to build and repair our bodies. Man is beginning to realize that foods grown organically, that is using natural, organic fertilizers without the use of chemicals, pesticides, or fungicides, will replenish the precious minerals and trace elements of the soil. A fruit, vegetable, grain, bean, or nut is only as nutritious as the soil it was grown in. **The nutrients of the soil eventually become part of the building blocks of our bodies.** Life can be measured in inches - inches of top soil! Eat organic fruits and vegetables whenever possible!

CHAPTER EIGHT

THE GENESIS DIET CONFIRMED

"You will know them by their fruits."
(Matthew 7:16)

Most people define what happens to them in their lives as "good luck" or "bad luck". Religious people call the good things that happen to them "blessings" and the bad things that happen to them "the devil". In both examples, the individuals are not taking responsibility for the results. But God's word says that "whatever a man sows, that he will also reap" (Galatians 6:7). So if you sow the causes of sickness, you will reap sickness and if you sow what supports health in your body, you will reap a healthy body.

The way a person lives, often referred to as **"a lifesyle"**, will produce certain predictable outcomes. A healthy lifestyle has the potential to produce such good fruit as a long, disease-free life, full of precious moments. An unhealthy lifestyle, which can be referred to as a **"deathstyle"**, most probably will produce bad fruit such as pain, suffering, illness, disease, and premature death.

The majority of Americans eat the Standard American Diet (S.A.D.) of high animal fats, refined sugars, and processed junk foods full of additives, chemicals, and pesticides. Add to this, drugs, alcohol, smoking, and caffeine (coffee, tea, soft drinks, and chocolate products) and you have the potential to develop many degenerative diseases. Half of all Americans will die of heart disease and another third will die of cancer. Forty percent of all Americans are overweight and it is common to develop arthritis and osteoporosis as we age. These are the statistical "fruits" of an unhealthy lifestyle.

God created our bodies to function best on His diet and according to His commandments and statutes. The dietary precepts of the Lord, outlined in the Scriptures, will bless **whosoever will** keep them. Today in other parts of the world, there are cultures that are virtually free of cancer, heart disease, strokes, diabetes, arthritis, PMS, and many other ailments that are considered common in America. These cultures that follow lifestyles proven to promote health should be the standard of wellness promoted by all doctors, nutritionists, and dieticians.

HEALTHY CULTURES

It seems logical to study people renowned for their superior health, longevity, and vitality. When studying the effects of foods on whole cultures, many times the negative effects are not fully seen in the first generation. It may take two or three generations for unhealthy food selections to harm the teeth, hair, bones, organs, and tissues of individuals in that culture. Truly, the nutritional sins of the parents are visited upon the third and fourth generations. And if there are cultures where generation after generation of the offspring remain disease-free, these people are showing good "fruits" and are worthy to ask, "What are they eating to stay well?"

Although scattered throughout the world, these cultures have strikingly similar eating and living patterns not only to each other, but also to the nutritional principles of the Bible. In many countries, the healthiest diet is simple and inexpensive. Often referred to as the "peasant diet" because it is based on what is considered the poor people's cuisine of grains, fruits, vegetables, and only a small amount of meat, fish, eggs, or dairy. This type of diet is low in fat and high in fiber with most of the calories coming from grains and legumes. We were commanded by the Lord to eat a lowfat, high complex carbohydrate diet and that is exactly what our genetic composition is designed to handle. These cultures confirm that **The Genesis Diet** is as valid today as when it was first given thousands of years ago. **God's principles of nutrition work for anyone, anywhere, that will follow them.**

Healthy Cultures

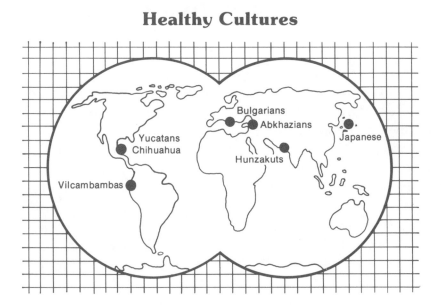

Such healthy cultures include the traditional Chinese and Japanese, the Vilcambambas of Ecuador, the Hunzakuts of Kashmir, the traditional Bulgarians, the Abkhazians of Georgian Russia, the Yucatan and Chihuahua Indians of Mexico and the Greek people from the island of Crete. Civilization and affluence bring with them the "king's delicacies" of high fat, refined sugars, and animal protein. As countries and cultures move from poverty to prosperity, infectious disease and malnutrition are replaced by the "diseases of civilization" - heart disease, cancer, diabetes, and obesity. Researchers are finding that a country's diet is intimately connected to the health of its people.

RESEARCH FROM AROUND THE WORLD

THE CHINESE STUDY

God's nutritional plan was confirmed by a recent study in China. From 1983 to 1988, the most comprehensive study ever done on diet and health was a joint effort involving Cornell University in the United States, the Chinese Academies of Preventative Medicine and Medical Sciences, and Oxford University in England. The nutritional study covered 6,500 Chinese adults from 65 representative counties and offered the researchers a unique opportunity to investigate the links between dietary practices, which vary greatly from region to region, and different types of diseases. The Chinese tend to spend their whole lives in the same location and eat the same kinds of locally grown foods their ancestors ate. Hundreds of food samples were taken and analyzed as well as individual blood screens and lifestyle information from participants.

The results of this in-depth nutritional study revealed how diet affects our health. One common nutritional myth in America is that obesity is directly related to the total number of calories consumed. It was once assumed that the body handled all calories in exactly the same way, but researchers now understand that there are three classes of calories: carbohydrates, fats, and proteins. Ninety-seven percent (97%) of all fat consumed is immediately stored as bodyfat (see **Breaking the Fat Barrier** for more information), whereas carbohydrates are more likely to be burned directly or stored as glycogen. This supports much recent evidence suggesting that dietary fat intake promotes obesity directly, rather than the total number of calories consumed. These facts explain why the Chinese, who consume 20% more calories per unit of body weight than Americans, are not suffering from obesity and heart problems. Also, they consume only 15-20% of their calories from fat whereas Americans consume 39%-43%.

The Chinese eat a plant-based diet consisting of carbohydrates and fiber that is scarce in fat and animal protein. It was once thought that too much fiber hinders the digestion and absorption of minerals, especially trace minerals such as iron.

Although the Chinese consume 34 grams of fiber per day as compared to only 11 grams per day for Americans, Chinese blood levels of zinc, iron, calcium, and magnesium are not compromised by the high fiber intake, nor are they lacking in iron. Even though their diets lack red meat, measurements taken on Chinese adults reveal excellent levels of iron.

American women are encouraged to increase their calcium intake in order to reduce the chances of osteoporosis. But in China, where the daily intake of calcium is half that consumed in the United States, there is little evidence of osteoporosis. Not only do the Chinese consume less calcium, but the calcium comes primarily from plant sources like leafy green vegetables and whole-grain cereals rather than animal sources like milk and cheese. How can a diet low in calcium and deficient in dairy products result in less osteoporosis? The answer lies in the protein intake of the two cultures. Americans consume 50% more protein daily than the Chinese and the greater the protein intake, the greater the loss of calcium!

High animal protein diets, like the one in America, increase the serum cholesterol levels. The average serum cholesterol level in the U.S. is 212 as compared with the Chinese average of only 125. High animal protein diets according to animal studies done at Cornell University, also promote the development of tumor growth and liver cancer.

One of the conclusions of this comprehensive six-year study is that Americans need to decrease their consumption of animal fat and animal protein in favor of dramatically increasing their consumption of plant-based foods—fruits, vegetables , and whole-grain cereals. The study suggests that increasing the consumption of plant foods will lessen the risks of various chronic degenerative diseases.

THE MEDITERRANEAN STUDY

The University of Minnesota School of Public Health released the results of a now famous study called the Seven Countries Study. They monitored the incidence of coronary heart disease in Finland, Greece, Italy, Japan, the Netherlands, the United States, and the former Yugoslavia. The study found that people living near the Mediterranean Sea had a very low rate of heart disease.

The study focused on villagers living on the Greek island of Crete whose heart disease rate was 90% lower than people living in the United States! Their diet was simple and consisted mainly of whole grain bread, olive oil, beans, nuts, vegetables, fruits, and small amounts of milk and cheese. They rarely consumed meat and ate fish only once a week. When meat was eaten, one pound fed six to eight people, and it was far leaner than U.S. feedlot beef. Only eight percent of the calories in the Cretan diet were from saturated fat, a reflection of their low intake of meat and dairy products.

This Seven Countries Study was one of the first large-scale epidemiological studies to establish a direct link between diet and heart disease. In 1991, the Harvard School of Public Health published an editorial in the New England Journal of Medicine endorsing what they called, "the Mediterranean diet" as a model for disease prevention. In a nutshell, foods from plant sources are the core of the Mediterranean diet, while foods from animal sources are used only sparingly.

Scientific research is beginning to "discover" what our Creator has always known and taught in His word. As we look at the nutritional similarities between these healthy cultures who live thousands of miles apart, we can see the stamp of Biblical nutrition all over their eating patterns.

OPTIMUM DIET FOR OPTIMUM HEALTH

Food	% IN DIET
1. Grains, Beans, Seeds, Nuts	50%
2. Vegetables	30%
3. Fruits	10%
4. Dairy Products	6%
5. Meat (Fish, fowl, beef, pork, lamb)	4%

Food Group	% IN DIET
1. Complex Carboyhdrates	70-75%
2. Fats	15-20%
3. Protein	10%

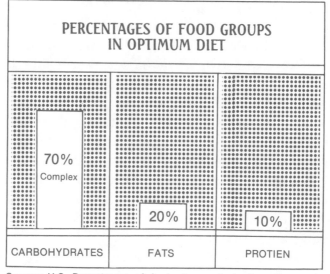

PERCENTAGES OF FOOD GROUPS IN OPTIMUM DIET

70%
Complex

20%

10%

CARBOHYDRATES | FATS | PROTIEN

Source: U.S. Department of Agriculture - Agriculture Research Service.

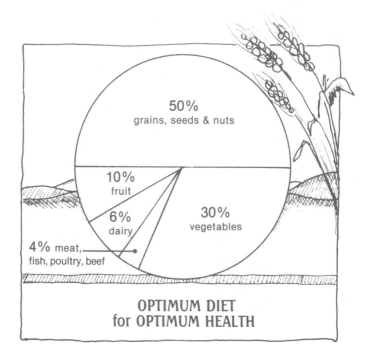

50%
grains, seeds & nuts

10%
fruit

6%
dairy

30%
vegetables

4% meat,
fish, poultry, beef

OPTIMUM DIET
for OPTIMUM HEALTH

THE LONGEVITY CULTURES

*"You shall therefore keep His statutes and
His commandments which I command you today,
that it may go well with you and your children
after you, and that you may prolong
your days in the land...."*
(Deuteronomy 4:40)

Many of the people in these extraordinary cultures
(shown on map on page 151) live over a hundred years in
good health! The average age is between 85-90 years old
with little degenerative disease; degenerative diseases
which we in America expect to develop as we age.

Comprehensive studies like the one in China, as well
as vital statistics and animals studies, are useful in determining nutritional information for a long, healthy life. It
is also valuable to study the foods of healthy cultures and
how they line up with the Word of God. But nothing is
more interesting than reading the personal testimonies
from some of these centenarians. These personal comments from people who have achieved the age of 100 or
more years come from Dr. Paavo Airola's book, <u>Worldwide
Secrets for Staying Young</u>. Dr. Airola spoke to them
personally and makes this observation:

> "While in Russia, I met several centenarians and
> discovered they had a few things in common. They
> were all moderate eaters, spent lots of time working
> outside, all were slim, all were poor, and all were
> happy! As far as their diet they either were total
> vegetarians or ate only very little meat."

One of the men Dr. Airola interviewed was 126 years old who gave him this testimony. This man outlived four wives!

> "I've worked hard all my life, but never had much money to worry about. I walk at least 5 miles every day, and ride a horse. I eat very little, and only when hungry——I never eat at regular times, but just when I feel really hungry. I was married four times, each time to a younger wife. Maybe this has helped me to stay young!"

The Russian Minister of Health told Dr. Airola that he had asked a centenarian of 146 years old from the Caucasus his secret for long life and this was his reply:

> "I've never had a boss over me. I have never been envious of what others have. And I periodically rejuvenated myself by marrying three times!"

It is truly refreshing to hear these testimonies for marriage in an age when 50% of most marriages end in divorce. These men were healthy, happy, and sexually active throughout their lives! The family life favors good health!

Mustafa Tasci was a vegetarian, never smoked or drank alcohol, walked a mile and a half each day, and he worked in his orchard. He was a Turkish man who was 144 years old, remarried at 83 when his first wife died and had 13 children and 50 grandchildren. Mustafa's secret of a long life was:

> "Eat moderately; stay away from meat, smoke, and alcohol; work every day; and surround yourself with young children."

Shirali Mislimov was the oldest man that Dr. Airola ever met. He was 166 years old and lived in the mountains of Abkhazia in Georgia (Russia). He was married three times. He fathered 23 children and he outlived all but two of them. His third wife was a hundred and seven years old and was healthy also. He believed in family life. These are his words about his life:

> "I was never in a hurry in my life, and I'm in no hurry to die now. There are two sources of long life: One is the gift of nature, and it is the pure air and clear water of the mountains, the fruit of the earth, peace, rest, and the soft warm climate of the highlands. The second source is within us. He lives long who enjoys life and bears no jealousy of others, whose heart harbors no malice or anger, who sings a lot and crys a little, who rises and retires with the sun, who likes to work, and who knows how to rest."

Another Abkhazian Dr. Airola met was a 104 year old superb horseman who offered these words of encouragement:

> "I've had 3 wives, I have 17 children, 48 grandchildren, and many great and great-great-grandchildren. I am loved and respected by all of them, and I have much to live for. I have never had many possessions. I always worked for others, and I have never been jealous of what others have. I go to sleep with the sun, and get up with the sun. I eat simple things, and only when I am really hungry. I never smoked, and I taste a little wine on festive occasions. I love these mountains and the sheep and my horse, and I sing throughout most of the day. Life is wonderful when you can enjoy good health...."

CONCLUSION: HEALTHY CULTURES

Dr. Airola said this about people who lived long lives: "In my studies of people who lived extraordinarily long lives in various parts of the world, I have found in addition to all the factors, such as sound nutrition of simple, unadulterated foods, scanty eating, poison-free environment, and plenty of exercise, they all possessed an inward calm. They were contented, happy with their families, neighbors, and the other villagers. This sense of importance, of being useful, having the respect and adoration of families and neighbors is an extremely important factor in longevity. Unfortunately, in the United States, oldsters usually face the opposite lot: they are excluded from a useful role in society, shoved into old peoples' homes, forgotten by families and relatives, feeling isolated, useless, and unloved."

America is a culture that worships youth rather than respects wisdom and old age. Perhaps that's one reason that America's citizens don't take better care of themselves. Who wants to be put aside when you are 65 years old, to live in isolation until you reach 100 years old! The cry today is "eat, drink, and be merry, for tomorrow you may die." Before the flood, at the time of Noah, people on the earth had that same attitude and God was not pleased with such a philosophy of life. The Lord desires for us to prosper, be in health, and live long upon the land. He also commands us to revere the aged and respect the wisdom that age can bring. God also said this about the "oldsters", as Dr. Airola called them:

"You shall rise before the gray headed and honor the presence of an old man, and fear your God: I am the Lord."

(Leviticus 19:32)

CHAPTER NINE

CHOOSE LIFE

"I have set before you life and death, blessing and cursing; therefore choose life, that both you and your descendants may live;"
(Deuteronomy 30:19)

Is life ours to choose? Ever since God placed Adam and Eve in the garden of Eden, the Lord has offered man two choices: following His ways which bring life or going our own way which ends in death. The two choices are before us, even as they were for the first man and woman. We can not expect health in our bodies while we continue to eat man-made foods that are pleasant to the eyes and pleasant to our perverted taste buds, but have no nutritional value. When we sow to our fleshly desires (appetite) in the food area, we will reap poor health and premature death. Mankind doesn't just "happen" to get sick; there is a cause for every effect. As the Scripture warns us:

"Do not be deceived, God is not mocked;
for whatever a man sows, that he will also reap.
For he who sows to his flesh
will of the flesh reap corruption..."
(Galatians 6:7-8)

Health is a choice that begins by setting your mind and heart upon the things above, where life and blessing dwell. Even though we have been banished from the Garden of Eden, we still have the **blueprint** in His word for eating **The Genesis Diet.** Moses and Caleb had God's blueprint. They both lived according to God's health principles, obeyed His word, and enjoyed long healthy lives into their "golden years". You will discover, as both Moses and Caleb did, that following God's dietary principles will help keep you healthy and strong in your old age.

MOSES

Moses lived at a time that the average age of most people was about the same as now - 70 years; yet Moses lived an additional 50 years! Although Moses lived 120 years, he exhibited no signs of advanced old age such as senility or physical degeneration. Instead, Moses retained his vitality until the day he died. He is indeed a testimony of divine health:

"Moses was a hundred and twenty years old when he died. His eyes were not dim nor his natural vigor abated (reduced)."

(Deuteronomy 34:7)

Moses did not die **from** old age, he died **in** old age. He completed his work for the Lord and God took him. Moses died healthy! How many Americans die healthy?

CALEB

Caleb was one of two faithful witnesses who gave a good report to Moses about the Promised Land. Joshua and Caleb were the only Israelites who left Egypt and entered the Promised Land over forty years later. Caleb gave a praise report of how the Lord kept him after leaving Egypt:

"And now, behold, the Lord has kept me alive,

as He said, these forty-five years....and now,

here I am this day, eighty-five years old."

(Joshua 14:10)

Caleb is not only thankful to God for keeping him alive to reach the ripe old age of eighty-five, but he continued his praise report by saying that he was just as healthy at eighty-five as he was at forty:

"As yet I am as strong this day as I was on the day

that Moses sent me, just as my strength was then,

so now is my strength for war, both for

going out and coming in."

(Joshua 14:11)

How many eighty-five year old men do you know who would be fit to do hand-to-hand combat with a sword? Caleb at eighty-five was just as strong and fit as when he was forty. Caleb was given as an inheritance, Mt. Hebron, which was protected by the Anakim, descendants of giants who were mighty men of war. But Caleb was a mighty man of faith:

"Now therefore, give me this mountain....for you

heard in that day how the Anakim were there....

It may be that the Lord will be with me, and I

shall be able to drive them out as the Lord said."

(Joshua 14:12)

The Bible makes it clear that faith without works is dead (James 2:17). Caleb was not only a hearer of the commandments and statutes of God, he was obedient to do God's word as Joshua testifies:

"And Joshua blessed him and gave Hebron to Caleb.......because he wholly followed the Lord God of Israel."
(Joshua 14:13-14)

Today, healthy cultures from all over the world follow the same **blueprint for health** that Moses and Caleb followed—the nutritional guidelines set forth by God in Genesis 1:29. They eat a diet primarily consisting of grains, beans, nuts, seeds, fruits, and vegetables (90% of diet) and only a little of the clean meats, poultry, and fish listed in Leviticus 11 and Deuteronomy 14.

The warning in Leviticus 3:16-17 to stay away from animal fats is echoed by recent scientific research. This research has come as a results of eating all the "king's delicacies" and now we are getting all the king's diseases—heart disease, strokes, cancer, arthritis, diabetes, and obesity. The Bible speaks to us about the curses that will come on all those who leave God's wisdom and choose the wisdom of the world:

" If you do not carefully observe all the words of this law.........then the Lord will bring upon you and your descendants extraordinary plagues— great and prolonged plagues—and serious and prolonged sicknesses..... Also every sickness and

every plague which is not written in the book
of the law, will the Lord bring upon you
until you are destroyed."
(Deuteronomy 28:58,59,61)

Could we be witnessing in our time the fulfillment of this prophesy spoken 3,500 years ago. Certainly such statistics as one out of every two of us will die of a heart attack or stroke and one out of every three of us will die from cancer are "great and prolonged plagues — serious and prolonged sicknesses — not written in the book...". But you still have time to choose to eat God's way and receive the promises that accompany obedience.

We are able, by the Spirit of God, who is within us, to renew our minds and choose the healthy life God has prepared for those who love Him.

"And do not be conformed to this world, but be
transformed by the renewing of your mind,
that you may prove what is the good and
acceptable and perfect will of God."
(Romans 12:2)

Speaking aloud the following proclamation helps renew your mind to the Word of God by confirming that your body is a temple of God:

My body is a temple for the Holy Spirit, re-
deemed, cleansed, and sanctified by the Blood
of Jesus. My members, the parts of my body,
are instruments of righteousness, yielded to
God for His service and for His glory. The devil
has no place in me, no power over me, no un-

settled claims against me. All has been settled
by the Blood of Jesus. I overcome Satan by the
Blood of the Lamb and by the word of my testimony, and I love not my life unto the death.
My body is for the Lord and the Lord is for my
body.*   Amen

LITTLE BY LITTLE

*"I will not drive them out from before you in one
year, lest the land become desolate and the beast of
the field become too numerous for you. Little by
little I will drive them out from before you, until
you have increased, and you inherit the land."*
(Exodus 23:30)

When the Lord delivered the children of Israel out of
Egypt He tested them in the wilderness to see what was
in their hearts. He didn't take them immediately into the
land "flowing with milk and honey". He prepared them by
trials, and these various trials tested their faith in God.
Only two, Joshua and Caleb, from the original two million
who left the "land of bondage", were permitted by the
Lord to enter the Promised Land. Joshua and Caleb were
truly "one in a million" men who believed God!
Do you believe God's word? Are you one in a million
who have been through many trials with your health, and
yet still believe God's word, " I am the Lord, your Healer."
Your faith has led you to read **The Genesis Diet** in hopes
of receiving an answer from God. Perhaps you have been
seeking answers for forty years and still have not lost
hope as Joshua and Caleb had not lost hope after forty

years in the wilderness. God's word has the answers. In fact, He is the answer!

Now it's time for you to enter your Promised Land of divine health. Although the children of Israel were promised this land and they entered by faith, battles were ahead for them. And so there are battles ahead for you. And even though the battle belongs to the Lord, you are required to pick up your sword, the Word of God, and fight.

God told the Israelites not to expect instant success in this new land, but victory would eventually, "little by little," be theirs. Victory would not be all at once; not even in a year! But little by little they would increase taking the land which God had promised them. They would increase in strength, in maturity, in wisdom, and most of all, they would increase in faith that God was with them in every battle. And so it will be for you. Believe and persevere in what God has said about divine health and He will give you the victory. It may not be in the first year, but you will find a level of health you never thought possible.

GOD'S FOODS BRING CHANGES

When you begin to eat God's foods, one of the changes you may experience is a feeling of weakness. As the body removes the poisons from the tissues, the heart begins to slow down and a "letdown" follows. This initial letdown lasts about ten days or longer and is followed by an increase of strength and greater well being. Be encouraged, your body needs a chance to adjust and complete its first phase of healing—**detoxification.** So rest and sleep as much as you can. The amount of accumulated toxins determines how long this phase will last. Be patient and thank God for the eventual victory.

During detoxification, your body is using its energies to do some needed "house cleaning". In short, the healing foods of God in this first phase of your physical restoration remove the garbage deposited in all the tissues. Cold or flu-like symptoms are common as the body cleanses the tissues and organs of unwanted "debris", as we discussed in the fasting chapter. Some people experience little or no symptoms, while others wonder if they are "getting sick". You may be eating well and still these symptoms occur. If such cleansing needs to happen in your body, remember that God will protect, sustain, deliver, heal, and restore you as you allow Him to help you through every battle. This is part of pulling down the stronghold of sickness and disease in your life. Choosing to follow God's nutritional guidelines is one step out of the harmful lifestyle practiced by many in the world today.

"And I heard a voice saying, Come out of her, my people, lest you share in her sins, and lest you receive of her plagues."
(Revelation 18:4)

Divine health is the birthright of all who believe and obey the Word of God. We can regain the health and vitality our Father in Heaven intended for us as we choose life. One way we do this is by eating the foods God has given to us. These good foods will help to renew our strength.

"Who satisfies your mouth with good things, So your youth is renewed like the eagle's."
(Psalm 103:5)

HE SENT HIS WORD

"He sent His word and healed them, And delivered them from their destructions."
(Psalm 107:20)

No matter how overweight you may be or sick and tired you feel, God's word can restore you. The following are a few testimonies of people just like you. These people, with the help of the Holy Spirit, have started eating **The Genesis Diet** and in a short time have received great benefits.

Dr. Tessler,
I want you to know that I took Genesis1:29 of God's word to stand on as a reminder of what He wanted for me to eat. Everytime I would weaken, I'd go back to the Word over and over again. God miraculously took away the desires for the wrong foods and would give me a hunger for more vegetables and fruits. I have lost 35 pounds and only have 10 more pounds to go! I have become a witness when people ask me how I lost weight.
Sincerely,
Liz from Montana

Dear Dr. Tessler,
I want to thank you and your wife, Laura, for your coobook, **Cooking for Life,** and **The Genesis Diet**. They are outstanding books. The greatest thing about eating this way is the endless adventure possible in combining grains and vegetables in tasty ways. It is so different because your emphasis is on what you can eat and not on what you can't eat. God sends us what we need, when we need it. I was certainly in need of a good nutritional

program when I heard of **The Genesis Diet.**
Love in Christ,
Bess from North Carolina

Dear Dr. Tessler,
I wanted to thank you for this wonderful life-saving health plan. I don't call it a diet plan at all, it taught me how to eat correctly. I have had serious health problems in the past like gallbladder, stomach, and colon problems. Not only do I no longer need stomach medicine, I have lost 34 pounds in three months! My stomach doesn't swell and hurt anymore. I praise God everyday for my health!
Yours very sincerely,
Margie from Missouri

P.S. Thank for all the wonderful recipes in **<u>Cooking for Life.</u>**

Dear Dr. Tessler,
I just wanted to drop you a note to tell you how terrific I feel! I have so much more energy than I use to. I feel God led me to His dietary plan. Praise God for that. I love the grains! I thank God for them each time I sit down to eat them. I really enjoy cooking this way. It's great fun!
Sincerely,
Judy from California

Dear Dr. Tessler,
<u>The Genesis Diet</u> made absolute sense from the moment I read the material. The diet is based on Godly principles. I have enjoyed the recommended foods and have felt not only satisfied and full, but energetic as well.

I truly feel that I have a new lease on life. I feel so good I don't want to sit around anymore. I have lost 32 pounds and my husband has lost over 45 pounds and our two daughters (ages 12 and 7) eat this way as well. We are all experiencing greater health God's way.

Sincerely,

Christen from Ohio

Dear Dr. Tessler,

My husband and I are using **The Genesis Diet** and the learning process is going well. I was delighted and surprised when a sleeping problem of six years duration was resolved. I now wake refreshed and I can accomplish more at home and at work. WOW! The welcome rest improved my attitude. My success has impressed the staff members of the residential school where I work.

Sincerely,

Doris from Kentucky

Dear Dr. Tessler,

Approximately five months into my pregnancy I began **The Genesis Diet.** Since this was my fourth pregnancy I was apprehensive about changing my diet. As my family and I began to implement **The Genesis Diet** into our life, we realized that it wasn't another "diet", but truly a lifestyle of great eating habits based upon God's word. As a mother of four and constantly on the go, I found this program to be a key. I showed no weight gain at each prenatal visit, yet the baby continued to show growth. Our baby was born at home, weighing 9 pounds and 12 ounces!

We give God the glory for such a blessed birth and healthy baby. Thank you for taking the time to search God's word and finding such relevant truths about nutrition.

Sincerely,

Lisa from Oklahoma

Dear Dr. Tessler,

My wife and I were on our way to Richmond, Virginia to watch our son play baseball on a Saturday afternoon when I heard you on the radio talking about **The Genesis Diet**. Since I am a preacher and you were talking about the Bible, I decided to listen. After ordering your books, **The Genesis Diet, Breaking the Fat Barrier,** and **Cooking for Life**, we started making changes. I started the plan at a weight of 267 pounds and my blood pressure was very high also. I lost 47 pounds in a little over three months and cut my blood pressure medicine more than in half! I want to say thank you, Dr. Tessler for a whole new life - a life filled with excitement and good health.

Sincerely,

Rev. Robert from Virginia

These dedicated people are no different than you are. They are ordinary people following an **extraordinary** God. They are mothers and fathers, husbands and wives, young and old, black and white, overweight and underweight. Most of them lead very busy lives, but they are not too busy to obey the instructions of their God for divine health. As you start eating **The Genesis Diet,** please write and share your testimony of how God's health principles are improving your life. Write to:

Dr. Gordon Tessler
P.O. Box 99005
Raleigh, North Carolina 27624

A CALL FROM HIM

For those of you who have read this book and are wondering if Jesus could really be the Messiah of the world, able to forgive your sins, and make you a new person, simply ask Him right now to reveal Himself to you personally. God so loved you that He permitted His only Son, the Messiah, to be brutally beaten and cruelly murdered on a tree for you. If there was any other way for you to have attained salvation, do you think God would have subjected Jesus to such degradation and unbearable pain?

Ask Jesus to come into your heart and to forgive you. The supernatural forgiveness He offers will permit you to experience His cleansing power and His exceedingly abundant love. With all your heart, repeat aloud this Miracle Prayer:

Lord Jesus, I come before you, just as I am. I am sorry for my sins, I repent of my sins, please forgive me. In your Name, I forgive all others for what they have done against me. I renounce the evil in my life. I give you my entire self - body, soul, and spirit. Lord Jesus, now and forever, I invite you into my life. Jesus, I accept you as my Lord and my Savior. Heal me, change me, strengthen me.

Thank you Lord Jesus for covering me with your precious blood. Come now and fill me with your Holy Spirit. I love You. I praise you Jesus. I thank you Jesus. I will follow you every day of my life. Amen.

If you have said this prayer, your past has been forgiven, no matter what you have done. Now you have a hope and a future! When circumstances and people try to convince you that you haven't changed, remember, **Jesus died for you**, that you may have a new life in Him. Whose report are you going to believe, theirs or His? God's word promises you a new beginning:

"Therefore, if anyone is in Christ, he is a new creation; old things have passed away; behold, all things have become new."
(II Corinthians 5:17)

*I Corinthians 6:19, Ephesians 1:7, Psalm 107:2, I John 1:7, Hebrews 13:12, Romans 6:13, Romans 8:33-34, Revelation 12:11, I Corinthians 6:13—Courtesy of the Derek Prince Ministries-International, P.O. Box 19501, Charlotte, North Carolina 28219-9501, USA

Be Well Publications

Dr. Gordon Tessler
P.O. Box 99005 • Raleigh, N.C. 27624 • (919) 870-9080

Lazy Person's Guide to Better Nutrition ($9.95 plus S/H)

This practical guide to better nutrition is simple to read and easy to understand. Through it you will learn that nutrition is the most natural and effective form of restoring and retaining your health. (132 pgs. with illustrations)

Topics Include:
- Increasing your energy • Controlling allergies • Reducing stress
- Taking supplements safely • Kicking the sugar habit and many more

Breaking the Fat Barrier ($12.95 plus S/H)

A book that tells you everything you need to know about dieting. (145 pages)

Topics Include:
- Expose the myths about dieting • Explains scientifically why diets fail
- Step-by-step approach to losing unwanted fat
- Lose weight without counting calories or starving
- Eat the foods that speed up your metabolism
- Eleven simple exercises to burn fat (illustrated)

Cooking for Life ($14.95 plus S/H)

Dr. Tessler and his wife, Laura, collaborate to make this Biblically-based cookbook fun for the whole family.

Topics Include:
- Over 200 delicious, easy to prepare, lowfat and nonfat recipes
- Four weeks of menu ideas
- Gives cholesterol, fat, fiber, protein, carbohydrate, sodium and calories for each recipe
- * The perfect companion for the *Lazy Person's Guide to Better Nutrition, Breaking the Fat Barrier, or The Genisis Diet*

The Genesis Diet ($12.95 plus S/H)

Table of Contents

Chapter I. Deceptive Foods	Chapter VI. Fasting for Health
Chapter II. Back To The Garden	Chapter VII. God's Pharmacy (Herbs)
Chapter III. Beyond The Garden	Chapter VIII. The Genesis Diet confirmed
Chapter IV. All The Fat Is The Lord's	Chapter IX. Choose Life
Chapter V. Did God Change His Mind?	

The Genesis Diet lays the Biblical foundation for optimum nutrition. The Lord has given us His nutritional plan so that we may walk in divine health and fulfill all of God's purposes for our lives.

Eating God's Way (Video) ($19.95 plus S/H)

In this 60 minute teaching video. Dr. Tessler outlines the Biblical principles for optimum nutrition. Taped before a live audience. Dr. Tessler's compelling and sometimes humorous presentation includes a question and answer time.

Train Up A Child (Video) ($19.95 plus S/H)

Parents are responsible for training up children spiritually, morally and nutritionally. This 2-part video begins with a Biblical teaching by Dr. Tessler on children's nutrition (Part I, 40 minutes) and includes another segment featuring Laura and Gordon Tessler demonstrating what to serve children for breakfast, lunch, dinner and snacks. (Part II, 45 minutes)

Get the *GREEN ADVANTAGE* ™

"The Good Greens"

"And the earth brought forth grass, the herb that yields seed according to its kind, and the tree that yields fruit, whose seed is in itself according to its kind. And God saw that it was good."

—GENESIS 1:12

VEGETABLE NUTRITION FOR THE WHOLE FAMILY

Dr. Tessler is committed to providing the finest concentrated vegetable nutrition available. One tablespoon of **Green Advantage™** provides the nutritional equivalent of 3 servings of green vegetables or 3 dark green leafy salads. With this organic vegetable powder you can be certain your body is receiving the power, energy and protection of green vegetables.

Green Advantage™

Ingredients per 3 tsp (1 tbsp)
Servings Per Bottle 30

Whole Leaf Green Grasses	
Barley Grass Powder	1500 mg
Wheat Grass Powder	1000 mg
Alfalfa Grass Powder	667 mg

Greens From The Sea	
Spirulina	600 mg
Chorella	200 mg
D. Salina	30 mg

Greens From The Land	
Spinach Powder	100 mg
Nettles Powder	100 mg
Dandelion Powder	97 mg
Beet Juice Powder	67 mg

Other Important Products	
Lecithin	1500 mg
Pectin	1300 mg
Barley Malt	650 mg
Brown Rice Bran	650 mg
Licorice	40 mg

Contains no added yeast, sugars, salt, egg, fats, flavors, gluten, dairy products, or preservatives. Nitrogen-Packed to remove corrosive oxygen. Store in refrigerator if not used within 6 weeks after opening.

Our barley and wheat cereal grasses are nutritionally concentrated vegetables grown in rich, organic soils that are herbicide and pesticide free. The alfalfa and red beet juice powder in **Green Advantage™** are also grown with the same care as the barley and wheat. Our sea vegetables like chlorella, spirulina and dunaliella salina, are selected for their purity and nutritional content from nations around the world.

B-Supreme

Get 100% of the Important B-Complex Vitamins Plus C

Vital for energy, B-Complex vitamins are involved in nearly every reaction in your body, from manufacturing of new red blood cells to the metabolism of carbohydrates, fat and protein. Unfortunately, modern day stresses of life can cause deficiencies of one or more of these B vitamins. Also, cooking and food processing destroys these precious vitamins.

B-Supreme is easy to take, fast acting, yeast and sodium free, contains no sugar, preservatives or sorbitol. **B-Supreme** dissolves under your tongue to enter your system in minutes, delivering 100% of your daily recommended allowance for B-Complex vitamins and vitamin C. A 30-day supply is only **$13.95 plus $3** shipping and handling and each sublingual tablet is individually packaged.

Since B-Complex vitamins and vitamin C are essential for energy, circulation, nerves, and metabolism and since these important vitamins are essential to everyone everyday, why not order your **B-Supreme today!**

B-Smart by taking B-Supreme

ORDER FORM

Description of Item	Qty.	Price	Total
Lazy Person's Guide to Better Nutrition		$ 9.95	
Breaking The Fat Barrier		$ 12.95	
Cooking For Life		$ 14.95	
The Genesis Diet		$ 12.95	
Eating God's Way (Video)		$ 19.95	
Train Up A Child (Video)		$ 19.95	
Green Advantage™ One Month Supply		$ 34.95	
Green Advantage™ Three Month Supply SAVE $15.00		$ 89.95	
*Green Advantage™ Automatic Reorder Plan (Credit Card Only) SAVE $5.00		$ 29.95	
B-Supreme		$ 13.95	
*B-Supreme Automatic Reorder Plan (Credit Card Only) SAVE $1.00		$ 12.95	

SHIPPING AND HANDLING	
Green Advantage (only) .... add $3 (ea.) **B-Supreme (only)** .... add $3 (ea.) $ 0.00 to $15.00 .... add $4 $15.01 to $30.00 .... add $5 $30.01 to $45.00 .... add $6 $45.01 to $70.00 .... add $7 $70.01 to $90.00 .... add $9 Over $90.01 .... add 10% **Canada** .... double charges **Overseas** .... triple charges	**SUBTOTAL**
	N.C. Residents Add 6% Sales Tax
	Shipping & Handling (See chart on left)
	Thanks for your Order **TOTAL**

CREDIT CARD NUMBER ☐☐☐☐ ☐☐☐☐ ☐☐☐☐ ☐☐☐☐

VISA ☐   **Master Card** ☐   **Discover** ☐   **Expire Date** ☐☐ ☐☐

Signature _____

Address _____

City _____ **State** _____ **Zip** _____ **Phone # (_____)** _____

---

*Automatic Re-Order Plan: We charge your credit card and ship the product

automatically to your door at the beginning of each month. You may cancel at anytime.

All materials shipped first class or UPS. Allow 1 to 2 weeks for delivery.

Make checks payable to BE WELL PUBLICATIONS in American currency drawn on U.S. bank.